WEIGHT LOSS
WITH
ANY FOOD

This book teaches how to produce
weight loss *in the proper way - as a result of*
systematic and gradual **fat loss.**

Publisher: KINECOR Publishing, L.L.C.

Editor: Darcy Greenwald
Graphic designer: Daniela Rosio Ramirez
Photographers: Tom Lauhon, Josip Čorak,
                      Tomislav Smiljan, Joe Adamczyk,
                      Brent Kieft

ISBN-13: 978-0692238349
ISBN-10: 0692238344

OTHER PUBLICATIONS BY NEVEN ČORAK:

- *Fitness & Bodybuilding* (2001)
- *Basics of nutrition for sports and recreation* (2000)
- *Ljepota tijela by Neven Čorak* (1995)
  "Beautiful body by Neven Čorak"
- *Vitko i lijepo žensko tijelo* (1994)
  "Slim and beautiful woman's body"
- *Prehrana sportaša* (1993)
  "Nutrition for athletes"
- *Stop celulit* (1993)
  "Stop cellulite"
- *Ljepota tijela* (1992)
  "Beautiful Body"
- *Body Building for Everyone* (1992)

www.neven-corak.com

ACKNOWLEDGMENTS

Every book is the result of a team effort of many individuals; this book is no exception. I wholeheartedly want to express my sincere gratitude to all of you who helped along the way.

I owe a particular debt of gratitude to my close friend and mentor Joe Adamczyk. His countless honest and perceptive suggestions, at times relentlessly delivered despite my stubbornness, made this book a much better product.

Finally, I am grateful to Anna, Joseph and Raquel, for all the joy and inspiration only children can bring.

To Astra, Hektor, Casper, Copper and Ruby.

CONTENTS

FAT LOSS – YOUR WAY

Fat loss is like sex. In sex, we all aim for a happy ending, but how we get there varies greatly from one person to the next. The same goes for fat loss. There are more potentially effective fat loss programs out there than there are fingerprints on people who use them. To actually produce a happy ending, though, those fat loss programs have to be done right. One of my main messages is: don't get stuck on *what* you do for your fat loss, but focus instead on *how* you do it. This book will teach you how to do it right.

The principles in this book apply to the widest variety of readers, regardless of whether you wish to lose one or 100 pounds, whether you are man or woman, old or young. Think about this book as a universal owner's manual on fat loss. It provides facts about fatness and it provides the best methods for how to lose fat.

These methods are timeless, efficient, and they do not discriminate. They are simple, they follow the rules of nature and the idea of our original design. They have been proven over and over by thousands of men and women. They are great because they do not advocate for some weight loss product, but instead only teach cold facts and inspire common sense. These methods are not mine. They belong to no individual or corporation. They belong to the natural order of things, and I just put them together in this book to the best of my ability.

DO NOT FOLLOW

When I peruse books, watch TV, read magazines or listen to radio advertisements on fat loss, I find myself asking, "What are these people talking about? Aren't we all just talking about fat loss?" Yes we are, but the majority of what is out there presents fat loss in confusing and even deceptive ways to distract you so you do not see the frauds for what they are.

This book is not another endless science fair of biochemistry and nutrition. It is also not a carnival of three-and-a-half second exercise programs, fountain of youth menus, or other fat loss lies or promises. This book will provide practical, relevant information for you to use to lose fat. It is written from extensive, real life fat loss experience, not from someone's theoretical pondering. You will read the bare facts, the truth stripped down from myths, commercial propaganda and manipulations.

These simple and brutally efficient fat loss methods have been known for generations, but they are largely ignored for two reasons. First, for these methods to be effective, individuals using them have to take responsibility for their own actions and their own results. Not many people are willing to do this. Second, the multibillion dollar weight loss and mass media industries cannot make money on these principles because they are natural, accessible to everyone, and free.

In this book I will not give you *my* diet, *my* exercise program or *my* fat loss product. You do not need to blindly follow someone else to lose fat. One of many great differences between this book and the fat loss clutter out there is this: they give you their programs and menus and tell you to follow them. I give you the understanding of your natural design and tell you to follow your mind.

DO IT YOUR WAY

In this book I will give you what you need in order to have the power and freedom to design and then fully execute your own successful, personal fat loss program from scratch or, alternatively, adjust any existing fat loss program to fit your needs. The book will serve as a fat loss primer, a strong base upon which you can make any program successful. You will also learn how to scan any fat loss diet, exercise program or product for possible fraud, and easily determine what you want to reject or include for yourself.

The best diet or exercise is not the one you get from a popular book, internet site or friend. The best program is the one you properly design for yourself, and the one that can be adapted as necessary to your specific, changing needs. That is the kind of program you will be able to design after reading this book. To accomplish this you do not need any prior experience or specialized knowledge about nutrition, exercise or fat loss. If you read other books, I suggest you keep the rules and ideas from this book in mind. Some of the rules and ideas that you will read here may sound radical, but they are not. They are just truthful, simple and logical. What makes them seem radical is that you are used to hearing just the opposite.

YOUR CHOICES

When I consider buying a book, I randomly turn to five scattered pages and read one paragraph on each. If none of what I read says something valuable or penetrating in its message, I put the book back and keep looking. If you glance through this book to see its value, I cannot know if you are going to buy it or not. However, I do know if you read it, your perception of fat loss will change. You will have a clear vision of the truth and differentiate it from the fat loss rubbish piled all around us. Then, you'll face these choices:

1. You will know the truth, but still decide to deceive yourself with common myths and manipulations about fat loss.
2. You will know the truth, but decide not to lose fat because it takes more than you are willing to give.
3. You will know the truth, and annihilate fat successfully.

A friend of mine once said, "When you lie to people, you manipulate them into an altered perception of reality. You rob them of the opportunity to choose their own right course of action". This book tells you the truth about fat loss. What you do with the truth is your choice.

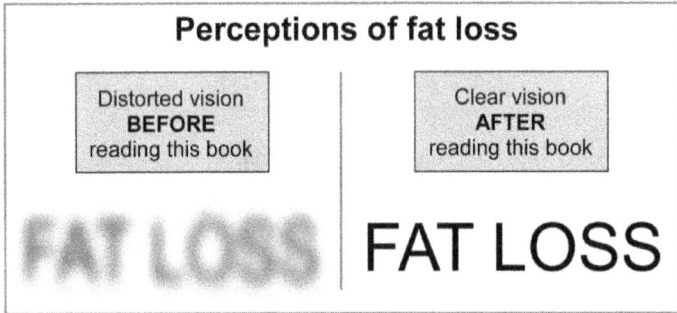

Perceptions of fat loss

Distorted vision **BEFORE** reading this book	Clear vision **AFTER** reading this book
FAT LOSS	**FAT LOSS**

GETTING THE MOST VALUE

Naturally, I would like you to read this book cover to cover, paying attention to each word, but realistically, that is not going to happen with every reader. We all have different ways we prefer to read a book, so read it your way. Here is some information about how this book is organized, as well as a few ideas I had in mind while I was writing.

I am not going to psych you up to lose fat. I am also not suggesting in any way that you are overly fat or that you should lose fat. That is and should be exclusively your decision. If you are indeed ready to do it, I will ultimately prepare you mentally and physically for the task ahead of you. This is the mission of this book.

PARDON MY LANGUAGE

In this book I primarily use the terms "fat" and "fatness", not for some derogatory reason, because there is nothing derogatory about being fat. I use it for accuracy and simplicity of communication. I don't think any good comes from sugar-coating the original term and switching to "large", "voluptuous", "big" or anything else. Some people react negatively to the terms "fat" or "fatness". This might indicate denial of reality and represent a serious mental obstacle on the way to fat loss. Detecting and overcoming these thoughts are necessary parts of successful fat loss. If this applies to you, you should perhaps start your fat loss with this as the very first step you take.

The book is divided into three sections. The introduction, "Fat loss – your way", gives you a general idea about the book and what you can expect. Eight chapters follow, and each has a short introduction at the beginning telling you about its contents. These eight chapters will teach you many facts and techniques about fat loss in real life that will make your fat loss easier and more efficient.

Appendix one, two and three are the last section of the book and they address exercise, nutrition and frequently asked questions. The appendices on exercise and nutrition are more theoretical, compared to the previous eight chapters. Even though they are more theoretical, they still contain plenty of practical advice and useful information for your day-to-day fat loss. Appendix three, Frequently Asked Questions, covers a wide range of topics related to fat loss. If you decide to read it first, it could give you an approximate idea about the contents of this book. It might even interest you in subjects you did not consider interesting before.

DON'T LET ME OFFEND YOU

Before this book was published, a friend of mine after proofreading this material told me, "Neven, I am afraid this book will offend many people. I don't think most people like to hear the truth". If you are one of those people, before you get offended by the truth, don't read any further. Put this book back on the shelf because it gives nothing but the bare truth. If you would rather read ridiculous lies, pick some other book on the fat loss subject; most of them promote nonsense and delusion, anyway.

Remember, this book is not another, "Don't think, just follow" fat loss sermon. It will teach you all you need to know about fat loss and then urge you to use it independently with audacity and clear thinking.

FOR BETTER
UNDERSTANDING

Units of energy – different reference materials display inconsistencies in units of energy that they use for food. Kilocalorie (kcal) is the measurement used to express the energy in food. One kilocalorie represents a thousand times more energy than a calorie (cal). In daily communication people typically say "calorie" when they are actually referring to "kilocalorie". Similarly, for simplicity in this book, the term calorie is used instead of kilocalorie. Also, some reference materials refer to food energy expressed in kilojoules (kJ). One kilocalorie equals 4.2 kilojoules.

Energy – in this book the term "energy" refers to the energy that the body needs, gets or spends for sustaining life functions and execution of daily activities. It also refers to the energy from energy-rich nutrients in food and drink (proteins, carbohydrates, fats and alcohol).

Energy-rich nutrients – one gram of protein releases about 4 calories, one gram of carbohydrates also releases about 4 calories, and one gram of fat releases about 9 calories. Additionally, one gram of alcohol releases about 7 calories.

Energy of human fat – I often refer to fat loss through energy deficit. One pound of human fat expressed in energy has approximately 3500 calories. Therefore, you have to create an energy deficit of 3500 calories to burn one pound of fat.

Units of mass – one ounce equals 28.3 grams, and one pound equals 453.6 grams (0.4536 kg). Approximately 2.2 pounds equals one kilogram.

RDA – stands for "Recommended Dietary Allowance" (sometimes referred to as "Recommended Daily Allowance"), the government-recommended daily amounts of nutrients sufficient to meet the requirements of over 95 percent of healthy adults. Such amounts are approximate and may vary according to specific circumstances such as growth, gender, pregnancy, lactation, health, level of physical activity and so on.

BMR – stands for "Basal Metabolic Rate", and is the daily amount of energy that the body needs while at rest in a neutrally temperate environment, with the digestive system being inactive (which requires about twelve hours of fasting). This energy is sufficient only for the functioning of the vital organs.

Lean Body Mass – represents the total mass of muscles, bones, organs and everything else in the body, except fat.

High Quality Proteins – also known as complete proteins, these are proteins that are suitable for satisfying our bodies' daily protein needs. They come from foods of animal origin, and should be present in our nutrition every day. On the other hand, low quality proteins (or incomplete proteins) are typically of plant origin, and are not suitable for satisfying our daily protein needs.

Resistance training – refers to exercising with free weights or resistance machines commonly used in fitness centers.

Cardio Training – also known as aerobic exercise, is used during fat loss for an accelerated fat burning process.

DISCLAIMER

Before applying any ideas, suggestions, programs or other information from this book, consult your physician to ensure that your plans will be beneficial to your health. Even though we all are designed in generally the same way, large or small individual differences exist, and they should be respected.

Especially if you have any health conditions (e.g. heart problems, diabetes) consult your physician, because some types of exercise or nutritional concepts may not be suitable for you. You want to lose fat, but also keep or even improve your health - otherwise it is not worth it!

***

The purpose of this book is to teach you how to lose excessive body fat in the most efficient and natural way. This book will enable you to do that regardless of what foods you eat.

Nevertheless, I want you to clearly understand my message. You absolutely should eat well-balanced and healthy nutrition. What kind of nutrition is well-balanced and healthy for your individual needs, is a decision you will have to make on your own or in cooperation with your physician and nutritionist. *This book is not designed to provide such advice.* Once you have chosen the type of nutrition best for you, this book will teach you how to adapt it to lose excessive body fat. By losing excessive body fat you should improve your health and well-being.

CHAPTER ONE

Right off the bat, Chapter One tells you to get off your couch, start your fat loss, and suck it up until you finish it. It delivers the importance of the mental side of fat loss and suggests ways to find and keep sufficient motivation until you reach your goal. It also delivers valuable guiding principles to make your expectations reasonable and fat loss program easier and more efficient.

THE MIND
A LIMITING FACTOR

I am absolutely certain that you will lose fat successfully if you follow the guidelines presented in this book. I don't have even the slightest doubt about that. These methods were brutally effective long before the Roman Empire, and they will be equally effective even after the US Government stops collecting taxes. Unfortunately, motivating you to start, and even more so to finish, is an entirely different story. Simply, fat loss is not possible without effective motivation. The body in its physical dimension is never the limiting factor. The body could, in fact, be considered the limiting factor if it had to endure starvation or unbearable exercise. However, in everyday reality, successful fat loss is achieved with a gradual approach over a prolonged period of time. A struggle for survival is not required. The body is not the reason you got fat in the first place, nor will it be the reason you cannot lose fat. Rather, the mind is guilty of both. For successful fat loss, the mind must set the clear course and resolutely lead the way, while the body obediently follows and executes its tasks.

> *The body is not the reason you got fat in the first place, nor will it be the reason you cannot lose fat. Rather, the mind is guilty of both.*

To be more precise regarding what I mean when I say the body or mind is a limiting factor during fat loss, I offer this explanation. If the body were a limiting factor, then even with the best motivation, intention and effort, you would not be able to continue either physical exercise or a diet. You would simply be either too exhausted, or nutritionally deprived. When this is not the case, your mind is sabotaging your progress by telling you to stop exercising or increase caloric intake.

THE INITIAL DECISION

Successful fat loss starts with the initial decision and motivation to lose fat. The motivation may arise from a wide range of needs and desires. Some will want to lose fat for health reasons, others for looks, love, hate, spite, work, sports, sex, or to prove a point. It is irrelevant what your motives are, as long as they are good enough for you. Many of my most motivated clients did not care about their health a bit, but started losing fat hoping to seduce the man or woman of their choice. Some may say that is a shallow reason. Maybe, but I believe being sufficiently motivated to take a first step is great; reasons leading to it do not matter much. Do not seek motivation from some "noble cause" or "perfect reason" if you do not have it at the moment. Use what you have as motivation to do the right thing and start moving toward your goal.

STAY THE COURSE

After you seize sufficient initial motivation and start your fat loss program, you must stay on course until you reach your goal. Every day thousands of people seize sufficient initial motivation and start their fat loss, but only a few will finish it. Again, that does not happen because of the body and physical limitations, but because of the mind and its destructive games. During fat loss the mind will often play games regarding food limitations, and occasionally regarding physical exercise.

Even during a mellow, physically easy-to-follow fat loss diet, you could experience a crisis due to a mind game, just because of the idea of having to limit your type and amount of food. Then, food often becomes a primary subject of thoughts. You may not even like a certain food, but the moment it becomes off limits, all of a sudden you desire it and want more and more of it. A good example is pizza for me. Before I started serious fat loss dieting, I did not care about pizza at all. Once I started dieting, I began craving pizza as if it had always been one of my favorite foods.

There is no genuine physical source for this desire for "forbidden fruits" in "forbidden amounts". The only real source is emotional craving, the mind playing a destructive game to ruin your fat loss. *This is the essential reason why people do not lose fat. The emotional desire arises, but there is not sufficient discipline to keep it restrained.* No one can completely eliminate all temptations and emotionally-based food cravings in a fat loss program, but with a proper approach much can be accomplished.

The fact is, the hungrier you get and the longer you persevere, not only emotional, but also physical food cravings will progressively arise until you answer them. This is our natural protection from starvation. To prevent or reduce such cravings, you should not expose yourself to fat loss programs that are too strict. This way you can at least eliminate physical if not emotional reasons for crises and possible outbreaks of overeating.

A SPOILED CHILD

When it comes to emotional food cravings, you should try to see them for what they really are. You can objectively evaluate if you are just being a spoiled child about something you want to eat, or if you really need it for an improved chance of fat loss success. Sometimes you may have to choose less appropriate foods (or exercises) in order to manage your mind and its cravings so you can proceed with your fat loss.

I am often asked while dieting why I eat white, refined rice, instead of nutritionally richer brown rice. The simple reason is because I like it better. The mental benefit for me of the better taste of the white rice outweighs by far the possible physiological benefit to my body coming from the brown rice. You must remember, if you manage your mind and avoid excessive mental crises, the rest is easy, a walk in the park, so to speak.

For that reason, during fat loss one of the tools I use to manage my mind is white rice. I like to overcook white rice and add diet sweeteners to it, making it look and taste like rice pudding. That is a meal I look forward to every time I diet. It does not sound like much when you think about it with a full stomach, but when tired and hungry, it becomes a delicious specialty. After all, hunger itself is by far the best spice.

Thus, "sweet, white, overcooked rice" for me is something I really need for an improved chance of fat loss success. It provides my mind with the satisfaction of a tasty food, while nutritional intake is still under control. However, if I let my daily desire for much better tasting cheesecake take over, that would be me letting my spoiled child side destroy my chance of fat loss success.

SHOOT HIM DOWN

My spoiled child side does not like to diet but does want cheesecake. After a prolonged period of dieting, self-control and "cheesecake craving", I can become a bit grumpy and dim down my easy going, charming personality. That is normal, and it happens to everyone. It may not happen at the beginning of your diet, or if you are not pushing too hard, but the minute you start to work hard on your fat loss, the chance of you becoming grumpy rapidly increases.

One of the world's best bodybuilders, Sergio Oliva, for some reason was shot by his ex-wife. At the beginning of my career when I was a young bodybuilder, I mentioned this to my mother, Mirjana. Quite a bit later, I was again on one of my competition diets, doing my usual thing. One day, seemingly out of the blue, she said, "Neven, I am not surprised that bodybuilder's ex-wife shot him. I am your mother so you do not have to worry, but when you get married, either stop bodybuilding, or make sure she does not have a gun." I gave her a blank look with an open mouth for a few moments, but after quick self-evaluation, I knew she was right.

BUY A SPORTS CAR

While "sweet, white, overcooked rice" can be one of the tools to prevent mental crises, preoccupying the mind with something other than food and thinking about your fat loss is an even more useful tool. Here is an example of an emotional fat loss crisis that was washed away just by redirecting my focus.

I was 24 and getting ready for the European championship in bodybuilding. I was consuming about 2000 calories per day and that was very low considering my body weight and level of training at the time. My diet was obviously strict and I was constantly thinking about food and days off. One day during my diet I went on a trip to Italy, about 150 miles away from Zagreb, my home town in Croatia. Unexpectedly I saw a sports car that I really liked. At that moment, I completely stopped thinking about food, as if I were not dieting at all. Over the course of the next three days while busy purchasing, importing, registering and showing off my new car, I was eating only 700-800 calories per day and not even noticing I was hungry or tired.

The point is, that the crisis I was experiencing was not caused by physical, but by mental reasons. When a more "important" subject took over

> *How can you fool yourself when the truth is staring you in the face?*

my thoughts, the crisis was gone. It was gone in spite of the fact that I was eating less than 50% of the previous amount of energy that had put me into crisis. Throughout my career I have had thousands of crises, but this was the first one that made me aware that the mind truly is the limiting factor during fat loss.

Rule number one: find something "important" (no matter how unimportant it may actually be) to preoccupy your mind during fat loss and you will have no problems pulling it off. For instance, most of my books were started during my diets. Writing helps me redirect my focus away from food.

Rule number two: if I had not carefully paid attention to the amount of food I consumed and recorded it in my fat loss journal, I would not have been able to draw these conclusions accurately. I would have probably thought I was not hungry anymore because I had eaten more while preoccupied with a new car. But when I saw the facts of 700 calories versus 2000 calories and no crisis, I felt embarrassed about my previous whining and complaining. If you decide to pay careful attention to what and how much you consume throughout the day by keeping a fat loss journal, your outlook on fatness and fat loss will change forever. You really cannot fool yourself when you know the truth.

GUN TO YOUR HEAD

Mental crises are more related to food limitations than exercise because, unlike with exercise, self-control regarding food is needed 24/7. However, when working with clients who start complaining that they are too tired to continue walking on a treadmill, for example, I urge them to analyze if they are just bored of walking or if they really are physically exhausted and must stop. I help them put things in perspective by asking, "If I had a gun to your head and told you I will kill you if you don't keep walking

> *When uncertain, exaggerate the actual circumstances to the extreme, and answers become crystal clear.*

for another six hours, would you stop now or keep walking?" I never heard anyone say "I would stop now"! By exaggerating the actual circumstances to the extreme, answers to our dilemmas become crystal clear.

MR. PRESIDENT

What must be done physically to lose fat is simple and clear beyond any doubt. However, for unmotivated individuals, finding sufficient motivation to first start and then maintain a proper fat loss program until it is finished is often "mission impossible". I wish I had a specific, repeatable solution for finding sufficient motivation. In attempts to motivate some of my clients, I have tried many things, producing more or less successful results. One of my longest and hardest searches for effective motivation ended in a very unexpected way. Here's the story.

I met my friend Tom in August 2008 when he came to me as a client wanting to lose fat. Though now retired, in his younger days Tom was a very successful college athlete. Later in life he advanced to become president of one of the largest electronics companies in the world, hence his nickname, "Mr. President". As with all of my fat loss clients, during the first hour or two with him I presented the fundamentals of losing fat. We then continued with training sessions of working out in a fitness center two to three times per week. Some sessions were tougher than others, but overall Tom was doing a very good job. In spite of hard work in the gym, his body weight did not drop a bit.

A few months later, still with the same body weight, Tom came to me obviously disturbed. On my inquiry, he replied that he could not lose weight no matter what he did because of a hormonal imbalance caused by a certain medical condition. I understood he had had surgery related to that problem a few years ago, and a hormonal imbalance was his reality. However, I tried to explain to him that in spite of his medical condition, he could still lose weight if he applied himself to a proper fat loss program.

Radical measures

After over an hour of talking, my usual explanations still did not penetrate the core of his depression and wrong convictions, so I decided to resort to radical measures. Conventional training sessions and diet programs were not enough, and something much more productive and specifically tailored to his needs had to be done. I asked him if he was willing to take a bet that I would help him lose 20 pounds in the next two weeks and prove him wrong – with the caveat that he would have to let me strictly control his nutrition and exercise. At first he fought the idea, but after I convinced him that all he could possibly lose was fat, he accepted my proposition. I also explained to him that I would expose him to an overly-strict fat loss program during those two weeks, which is not recommended for a lengthy period of time. It would, however, be suitable for a shorter time in order to make rapid progress and eliminate his disbeliefs and worries. This also means you as a reader of this book should be slower and more gradual with your fat loss than what I had Tom do.

That same afternoon we went together to acquire all the necessary supplies for his fat loss. Starting the next morning and for the next two weeks I went to his house at 8:30 to prepare his meals for the day. All meals were precisely measured and organized with an approximate schedule of consumption. We even designated one refrigerator exclusively for his food; I wanted to eliminate unnecessary temptation and keep him away from other foods that were not on his fat loss list. I was checking his fat loss journal daily for completeness of records and accuracy of calculations.

For physical exercise, we walked around a nearby lake and golf course twice a day at a slow to a moderate pace for about 90 minutes each time. We did not lift weights during those two weeks, but we did lunges, squats, pushups, abdominals, and similar exercises at intervals during our walks.

Needless to say, Tom lost more than 20 pounds in those two weeks. He even continued for another week, and during those three weeks he lowered his body weight by 31 pounds. When we started he was 316 pounds, and three weeks later he was 285. And yes, he still had a hormonal imbalance during those three weeks.

Back to 316

Unfortunately, this is not the end of the story. A few months later Tom welcomed back his usual 316 pounds and embraced them like they were a life line. During the next two years I tried everything I knew to motivate him to lose fat. I explained the facts again and again, warned him about his health, gave him emotional support, praised him, criticized him, insulted him, "reverse psychology-ed" him. I even wanted him to get actively involved in writing this book, hoping that would motivate him. The only thing I didn't try was physically beating him. I was not the only one trying. His personal physician, friends and family members were doing the same. Sadly, there were no signs of life, only radio silence between Ground Control and Major Tom. Now comes a rather shocking twist to the story.

Racquetball

Getting Tom to go to the gym was like pulling teeth. After two years, in our attempt to find a physical activity he would like and regularly use, Tom offered to teach me how to play racquetball. I accepted it gladly in spite of the fact that I had never played before, and Tom was an excellent player with decades of experience. As a result of this unequal skills ratio, it took me over 50 games of continuous and brutal defeats before I started winning. My improved racquetball skills would not have been enough if they were not generously helped by Tom's "morbidly obese" physical condition, as so eloquently described by his personal physician.

As I started winning, I could not resist making jokes and teasing Tom with overblown remarks about my new racquetball skills. He put up with it until one day he said, "I have had enough of your bragging. I am going to lose weight, and you will not score one more point". "WOW," I said, and teased him even more, not only about racquetball, but also about his unsuccessful fat loss attempts during the last two years. I was convinced that he would never be sufficiently motivated to lose fat, since even health problems related to obesity did not get him going. If that didn't do it, how could a few racquetball defeats make the difference?

Was I wrong in my judgment! After that, Tom committed to his fat loss more seriously than ever before, and as of this writing he is still successfully losing fat. How long this will last, I do not know, but currently it is working great. From all the strong reasons he had to lose fat, such a seemingly insignificant thing, hands down, out-powered them all. Human motivation really does work in mysterious ways.

MAKE IT EASIER
ON YOURSELF

If you decide to lose fat, use your motivation and hard work as efficiently as possible, and make it easier on yourself. Hopefully the following recommendations will help you avoid unnecessary effort, disappointment or wasted time.

DON'T MYSTIFY IT

When thinking about fat loss, don't mystify it. Fat loss is simple and natural; disregard myths and commercial manipulations.

FOLLOW YOUR
OWN MIND

When evaluating if you are too fat or not, make sure the conclusions are consistent with your genuine beliefs. Do not let others influence your thoughts about whether you are fat. Significant others, friends, celebrities, mass media or others may suggest you should look a certain way. Accept their suggestion only if it matches your best interests and your true beliefs.

WHAT ONE PERSON CAN DO,
ANOTHER CAN DO

Many people don't believe strongly enough in themselves, thinking they cannot reach their goals. You likely cannot run the world record for 100 meters, but you can run fast enough. We are brainwashed with implanted ideas of false limitations. Get rid of that junk immediately, believe in yourself, and believe that you can accomplish your goals, regarding fat loss or anything else. And you will.

DISREGARD
PAST FAILURES

If you have previous negative fat loss experiences (and who doesn't), do not project them onto these fat loss principles. Use concepts from this book and you will successfully annihilate fat. You will have a positive fat loss experience, regardless of how many times you failed before.

EVERYBODY
KNOWS SOMEBODY

It seems like everybody knows somebody who lost fat in some super-efficient, easy or exotic way that defied all rules of nature. No matter how convincing and charming it may sound, or what that person apparently did, it always comes down to the same bare truth. Exotic and foreign, or plain and domestic, a fat loss program will produce the intended result only if it obeys the ultimate law of fat loss.

ELBOW GREASE
AND MOTIVATION

Knowing what fatness is, knowing how to treat it, or knowing that it will be good for you to lose fat, are not enough. You must put some elbow grease to it, and for that you need motivation and will power. If at the moment your motivation and will power are not strong enough to follow your program, don't bother, because you will not reach your goal. Fatness is frustrating enough by itself; you do not need additional frustration caused by failed fat loss attempts. Do it when you are truly ready.

TAKE RESPONSIBILITY

Don't blame your fatness or your inability to lose fat on your body's genetics or your life circumstances. Don't just go through the motions of following someone else's fat loss program, romantically hoping it will suddenly produce results, while the facts show the only thing it is producing is wasted time. Don't go around telling people you are doing your best, while there is no sign that you are losing fat. Fat loss does not care about whether or not you are doing your best. Just do what it takes! Take responsibility for your fat loss, create a program that will work for you, and you will lose fat.

IT'S YOUR BUSINESS

When starting on a fat loss program, do not make it other people's business or responsibility. Your fat loss is your business. Keep it that way. Do not ask someone else to be on a diet with you. Do not ask others to prepare your diet food or not to have certain food in the refrigerator. Do not cling to your training partner to make it through your workout. Any help is welcome, but essentially you must be able to do it yourself, regardless of what others around you think, do or eat.

EASY ON GOALS
AND DEADLINES

Set a goal that is meaningful but also reasonable to you, and give yourself enough time to reach it. Don't rush your fat loss, take your time. By rushing it you will cause unneeded stress. If you have an imposed deadline, then start fat loss as early as possible. A few weeks too long is better than one day too short. When not pressed for time, fat loss is much easier, and results are better. Remember the saying "It is not important how fast you progress, as long as you keep progressing". Deadlines are great for accomplishing goals, but set them conservatively.

BEYOND NUMERIC GOALS

Many people set a particular body weight or body fat percentage as their fat loss goal. Sometimes people just imagine a body weight or body fat percentage that sounds "cool" to them without knowing how it will be for them in real life. Setting numbers could be a good start, and it is easier to reach your goal if it is precisely defined. But when you reach your "numbers", if you are still not happy with the result, you must continue. If you are happy before you have reached your initially desired numbers, stop then. In essence, the numbers are not important at all. How you feel, perform and look are the criteria you should follow.

ROLE MODELS

Role models are good guidelines for your goal, but do not try to mimic them exactly. That is basically impossible. We are all different, so respect your individual uniqueness. When you are done with your fat loss, don't be surprised if you end up looking even better than your initial role models. Then you could set new goals and maybe find new role models. However, your best self should be your only true role model.

SET SMALLER GOALS

Especially if your final goal is big, I suggest you break it down into smaller units. For instance, setting and achieving a fat loss goal of three pounds per week or even 15 pounds per month will be much more motivating and friendly than exclusively thinking about losing 150 pounds one year down the road. By achieving smaller goals, you create frequent feelings of success. These positive feelings will help keep you motivated on your way to the final goal.

WRITE IT – TALK ABOUT IT

Write your goal on a piece of paper. Then, look at it every day, and see how you are advancing toward your written promise. That will increase your awareness and make your goal become more real. If you want support, you could post your intentions and pictures on the Internet. Then, keep reporting about your fat loss progress.

TEMPER IT DOWN

Sometimes too much motivation can be as bad as not enough motivation. People occasionally start fat loss like there is no tomorrow because something greatly inspires them in the moment, but then, they burn out in a few days. Losing fat is not sprinting, but rather a long distance race. Temper down your motivation and desire, and use a reasonable program that you can endure long enough to reach your goal. In time you will learn how much you can push yourself without burning out. Until then, go easy on your fat loss, but keep going.

RAISE THE BAR,
ENJOY THE ACCOMPLISHMENT

We often raise the bar after accomplishing our previous goal. That is normal and welcome. However, sometimes that keeps us chasing satisfaction in new goals and stops us from enjoying the present moment. Don't let that slip out of control. Enjoy the present moment and what is already accomplished, even when you are still striving for better.

CONVERT BAD INTO GOOD

During your fat loss, life does not stop, and many things will happen. Some will be small, some big, some good and some bad. No matter what comes your way, use it to amplify your focus and efforts towards your goal. Train your mind to use absolutely anything as a forward driving force.

LASER OR LIGHT BULB

Don't let your focus be distracted from your fat loss. Compare a laser and a light bulb. They are both lights, but because of precise focus, a laser reaches much farther and points exactly to the target. If more power is put into the laser and its focused light beam, it will cut through everything that gets in the way of its target. When aiming for your goal, be a laser.

DON'T GIVE UP

Sometimes in life some people do get lucky and win more than they deserve. On the other hand, many never get what they deserve. Either way, by not giving up, your chances of success are drastically increased. Even better, if you keep following your fat loss program and do not give up, your fat loss success is guaranteed. No matter how corny it may sound, don't give up, and you will lose fat.

TWO WEEKS

When you start losing fat, especially if you decide to use an aggressive approach, it will take you some time to get used to it. In the beginning it can be pretty uncomfortable, but endure the first two weeks, and it will become easier, especially as you see obvious progress.

VANILLA AND CHOCOLATE

Fifty years ago we had two flavors of ice cream, vanilla and chocolate. Today we have hundreds of flavors, but basic vanilla and chocolate are still the most popular. When you compose your fat loss program, do the same. Stick with basic foods and exercises, and avoid trends, modern confusion and exaggerations. The simplicity of the basics is usually the most effective approach.

THINK AND GROW LEAN

The book "Think and Grow Rich" delivers many great messages, but the best one is probably in the title itself, think and you will grow rich. The same goes for fat loss. Think about what you want and think how it is achievable. Our thoughts almost always create our reality. Think logically and you will grow lean.

CHAPTER TWO

We ask ourselves, deeply puzzled, "Am I fat due to a hormonal imbalance, or is it viral after all?" while crunching on our buttered popcorn and devouring tooth-rotting candies. Wow, that's a hard one to figure out.

Sarcasm aside, Chapter Two illuminates undeniable laws regarding fatness and proper fat loss. It explains how to determine fatness and the factors influencing our body figure. It also eradicates the common, deeply ingrained misconception that weight loss equals fat loss. They are not the same.

WHAT'S UP WITH MY FIGURE?

Body figure is mostly determined by three factors, fatness being only one of them.

- Size and proportion of the skeleton
- Size and proportions of muscles
- Quantity and distribution of fat

Of the factors influencing the body figure, the contents of this book are focused on fatness and its treatment.

QUANTITY
AND DISTRIBUTION OF FAT

This factor has the strongest impact on the body figure and is influenced by genetics, but it is far more influenced by lifestyle, especially nutrition. There are two basic ways fat deposits can compromise one's look.

Proportional accumulation of fat

Proportional accumulation of fat on the body often does not look bad if fat deposits are not excessive. For example, if a person with smaller bone structure and smaller muscle mass proportionally accumulates a moderate amount of fat, the body figure may even improve, because it will not look too skinny any longer. Unfortunately, not all people accumulate fat proportionally, and even for those who do, there is a risk of excessive accumulation.

However, if a person has reached the desired body weight and volume by gaining fat proportionally and moderately, the body will still not look as hard, firm, defined and ripped as if the same weight or volume was achieved by muscle development. This is probably the strongest aesthetic issue with proportional and moderate fat accumulation.

Disproportional accumulation of fat

Disproportional accumulation of fat on the body, especially if excessive, can severely ruin a body figure, more than skeletal or muscular factors combined. Disproportional accumulation of fat usually happens either in the upper part of the body (chest and stomach), or in the lower half of the body, from the waist down (hips and legs).

WEIGHT LOSS VS. FAT LOSS

The difference between weight loss and fat loss is significant.

Weight loss

Weight loss refers only to the reduction of body weight, regardless of whether body weight was reduced by fat loss, loss of muscle, dehydration, cutting off hair, or any other reason. Weight loss could be completely unrelated to fat loss, even though there is a strong correlation between the two. For instance, a person can lose 20 pounds of muscle mass and, in addition, gain 10 pounds of fat. That person will weigh 10 pounds less but have 10 pounds more fat, which generally is not desirable. This is typical for athletes after an active sports career. They often weigh less but have more fat.

Fat loss

Fat loss refers precisely to the reduction of fat in the body composition and in most cases is accompanied by weight loss, but not always. Sometimes a person can reduce the amount of fat on the body and still have the same or even higher body weight than before. This can happen if a person first lost, for example, 10 pounds of fat, and then kept the fat off but later developed 10 pounds of muscle. This person will have the same body weight but less fat than before. This is the most likely scenario.

A less likely scenario is when a person develops muscle mass while at the same time losing fat. In this case, body weight stays the same because the gained pounds of muscle will compensate for lost pounds of fat. The person could keep (or even increase) body weight, in spite of the reduced amount of body fat.

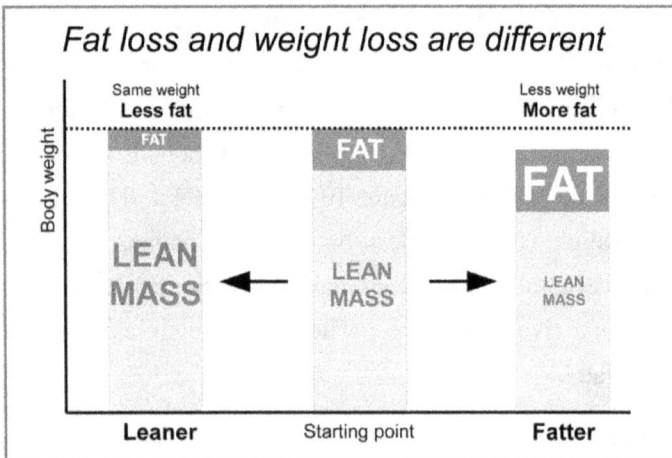

Fat loss and weight loss are different

Caution is needed. If you are on a fat loss program and not losing body weight, it is likely because your fat loss program is insufficient, not because you are developing muscles. Muscle development requires a different nutritional program than fat loss. Fat loss can be perceived as time at work, while muscle development is leisure time. They can overlap occasionally, but generally they do not go together.

FATNESS AND OBESITY

Fatness is an increased percentage of fat in the body's composition. Obesity is a term for excess body fat deposits to the extent that they may cause health problems. There are several categories that describe the percentage of fat in the body's composition. The exact names or values for these categories, and even the number of categories, vary from one source to another, but generally they are in the same ballpark.

Category	Women	Men
Essential Fat	up to 10%	up to 5%
Healthy Range	11–30%	6–25%
Obesity	31% and over	26% and over

The category "Essential Fat" represents the level of body fat under which you should not go. It is recommended that you do not go under 10% if you are a woman or 5% if you are a man. If you do, your health could be negatively affected. The category "Obesity" also represents possible health troubles, so keep your body fat in the "Healthy Range" category. As you get older, it is expected that your body fat percentage will increase by a few percentage points, but it should still stay within healthy ranges.

Let us say you are a woman weighing 150 pounds, and you have 20 percent body fat. What that means is that you have 120 pounds of lean body mass (bones, muscles, organs and other tissues), and on top of that you have an additional 30 pounds of fat (20% of 150 is 30 pounds). According to this table you are in the "Healthy Range" category, meaning that is a healthy body fat percentage for you.

If you gain an additional 30 pounds of fat, but maintain the same lean body mass of 120 pounds, then you would weigh 180 pounds. In this scenario you have 60 pounds of fat deposits on top of your lean body mass, and that is about 33% body fat. You are now in the "Obesity" category, and you should lose fat.

On the other hand, if you lost 20 pounds of fat, but maintained the same lean body mass of 120 pounds, then you would weigh 130 pounds. In this scenario you have 10 pounds of fat deposits on top of your lean body mass, and that is under 8% body fat. You are now in the "Essential Fat" category, and you should gain fat.

DETERMINING FATNESS

Putting obvious medical reasons and fitness criteria aside, being fat or not is purely a matter of personal perception. I have had clients feeling fat with very low body fat percentage (6%), while others thought their high body fat was actually muscle tissue and wanted even more of it. Differences in perception are truly amazing.

People use various subjective criteria to evaluate their fatness, including how they fit into clothes from their younger days; looking, feeling and performing a certain way; comparing themselves to other people; and so on. In addition to these subjective criteria, more "numeric" methods are available, and some are listed below.

Body weight

Body weight is the most common criteria, but not the best indicator of actual fatness. In most cases, there is a very strong correlation between body weight and degree of fat deposits. However, if you are a very muscular person, you will be heavy even if your body fat is very low. Muscle tissue weighs more than fat tissue, making a muscular person with smaller body volume weigh the same, or even more, than a fatter person with larger body volume. That is why some individuals (most commonly, athletes) with more muscle mass can be very heavy. They are not fat, though, because their increased body weight does not come from fat deposits. Rather, it comes from lean body mass which is mostly desirable in spite of increased body weight.

Therefore, measuring body weight alone can be misleading. When I was competing in bodybuilding, my training weight was about 315 pounds with only 9% body fat, according to one method using skin fold measurements. As I write this I am about 240 pounds with approximately 19% body fat. Now I have 10% more fat but 75 pounds less body weight than before. I am fatter even though much lighter due to the muscle loss.

To measure body weight correctly, you have to be as consistent as possible, otherwise results will be inaccurate. Always use the same scale, positioned on the same floor surface and in the same spot. Weigh yourself at the same time of day, with the same amount of food and drink consumed before weighing, and in the same type of clothing. Many people prefer weighing themselves in the morning, naked, on an empty stomach, after using the bathroom.

Body fat percentage

Body fat percentage is probably the best indicator of actual fatness. It tells you what percentage of your total body composition belongs to fat. Methods of measuring body fat percentage are not completely accurate. They are, more or less, precise guessing. It is still impossible to determine the exact body fat percentage for a living person.

As technology progresses, the number and accuracy of methods for measuring body fat percentage is increasing. My favorite still is using skin folds. It is a simple, widely used method, and requires a caliper that you can purchase for as low as $20. It gives fairly accurate results by taking into consideration primarily skin folds, but also gender, age, body weight and fitness level. Specifications may vary, but detailed instructions should be available with the caliper of your choice. Simplified, the thicker the skin folds you have, the fatter you are.

Don't worry that body fat percent measuring methods are not completely accurate. It is not really important if they missed by 1% or even 10% of the actual amount of fat in your body composition. Most important is that they are consistent in their accuracy or mistake. Then they are great indicators of positive or negative changes during a fat loss program. For them to show fat loss or gain correctly, measuring consistency is of utmost importance. A person must always use the same method, done with the same assistant, in the exact same way. Otherwise changes in results could be due to measuring inconsistencies rather than changes in body fat percentage. Before using a certain method, learn its specifications.

Also, if you are interested in achieving extremely low body fat results, be careful. You may hear others brag that they have dropped their body fat as low as only one or two percent. I once had a guy try to convince me he had zero body fat. I do not know anyone who has ever legitimately measured lower than 3% of body fat. I don't even know if any commonly used method could reliably measure anything so low. Therefore, do not try starving yourself to death in pursuit of someone's fairy-tale of "one percent" body fat or similar low results. I never measured my body fat percentage when competing at bodybuilding shows, because it is more important how your body looks on the stage than what percentage of body fat you have. However, I did measure my body fat percentage for some of my books and lectures, and for a few other reasons. The lowest I ever recorded my body fat by skin folds was 3.1%, and that was the equivalent of my prime conditioning while competing in bodybuilding (see page 58).

Body mass index (BMI)

Body mass index is an "outdated" measure of fatness. It correlates body weight and height. BMI is not accurate for people with exaggerated muscularity, individuals with increased body weight but low body fat percentage. Because of increased body weight when compared to height, BMI will incorrectly assume a high level of fatness.

Circumference measurements

Circumference measurements can be solid indicators of fatness, but much greater help in tracking fat loss progress. At the beginning, measure your body parts and then start losing fat. As you go, periodically recheck results. It is normal to notice different dynamics of change in circumference from one body part to another. For example, during the first month, your waist line could lose 5 inches, while your calves are still almost the same size. When I take my circumference measurements, I measure my neck, chest, waist, hips and upper arm, thigh and calf of the right or left side of my body. As with all other methods, consistency in taking measurements is needed here as well, otherwise results will be misleading.

Photos

Photos are more subjective criteria for determining fatness than previously described "numeric" methods, but they can be very helpful. People like to say they are not photogenic and don't look good in photos. The fact is you can appear better or worse in some photos, but generally photos show the cold fact of what stood in front of the camera.

A friend of mine made a very good point about how important photos can be for bringing you back to reality and showing actual fatness. He said he always knew he was getting fat, but only when he saw photos from a family birthday party did he truly realize what a "large" man he had become. Sometimes you can look in the mirror for years and not see facts as clearly as you will after just one brief look at a photo.

If you want before, during and after photos to show changes properly, they must all be taken in consistent conditions. The camera, position of the camera, lighting, your pose and clothing must be the same every time or you may see false changes. When you take photos of your physique for comparison, show as much of your naked body as comfortably possible. Drawing conclusions based on before and after pictures of a person who is mostly covered by clothing is equally as effective as determining if you prefer one wrapped Christmas present over another.

THE POINT IS,
WHO CARES ABOUT NUMBERS

My advice is to check body weight and circumference measurements since they are easily obtained, and optionally to check body fat percentage if a reliable method is available. These methods are solid indicators of fatness or fat loss progress, especially when combined together. However, photos, the mirror and your stamina walking up the stairs can sometimes be better indicators. Basically, who cares what your scale, tape-measure or caliper says. In essence, the results are nothing but numbers. What matters is how you feel, perform and look. However, numbers can be a great "eye-opener" showing you the measurable facts.

Who cares about the scale, tape-measure or caliper – focus on how you feel, perform and look.

WHAT MAKES US FAT?

Fat deposits are created from excessive, unused energy that has been consumed by eating or drinking. This is known as *energy surplus*, and it is the cause of fatness. There is no mystery. Everything else you hear related to fatness is simply more or less important circumstances that can only

> *Only one thing makes us fat – ENERGY SURPLUS.*

influence the balance between consumed and spent energy. But those circumstances will not make you fat if you are not in the state of energy surplus.

MORE IMPORTANT CIRCUMSTANCES

Here are the most important circumstances that can influence the balance between consumed and spent energy:

Nutrition

Nutrition (energy consumption) has by far the strongest impact on the degree of fatness. When looking for a cause of fatness, look no further. Even if you only regulate the energy level of your nutrition, you can roughly eliminate fatness.

Physical activity

Physical activity (energy expenditure) has the second strongest impact on the degree of fatness. However, it does not even come close to the influence of nutrition. In most cases, physical activity by itself will not be enough to produce fat loss because it cannot expend all the excessive energy that can easily be consumed. Physical activity together with an energy reduced diet will produce the best fat loss results.

LESS IMPORTANT CIRCUMSTANCES

Less important circumstances that can influence the balance between consumed and spent energy by influencing the body's energy expenditure include, but are not limited to, the following:

- Genetic heredity
- Certain medical conditions (for example, hormonal imbalance)
- Use of some medications

You can have one or even all of these less important circumstances, but the circumstances will not eliminate the body's energy needs. Circumstances will only either increase or decrease energy needs. The body will have energy needs as long as it is alive. Regardless of any circumstances, the bottom line is still the same. *Fatness will not happen if energy consumption is the same or lower than energy expenditure.* No matter how low your body's energy needs are, the choice to keep consumption and expenditure in proper balance and avoid entering the state of energy surplus is completely within your power.

Speaking of energy needs: we favor cars that need less energy to perform their duties (have "high gas mileage"). On the other hand, if our bodies need less energy we complain about it and call it "slow metabolism". Interestingly, high gas mileage vehicles and slow metabolism bodies both save us money by using less energy.

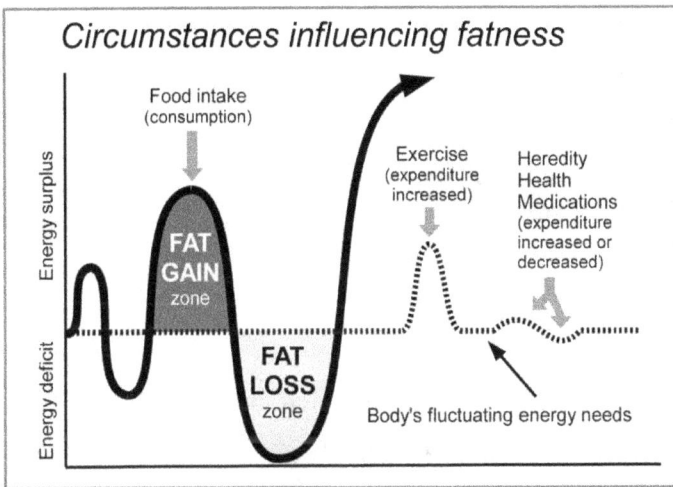

Circumstances influencing fatness

WHY DO WE STORE FAT?

Fat deposits are the energy reservoir of the human body, the body's "safety net". The body stores excessive energy in fat deposits so it can be used for survival in the future, when food may not be available. Instead of throwing it away now, the body saves it for later. Regardless if you have one or 100 pounds of fat deposits, the principle is the same. Similarly, toning, firming and defining your body all require compliance with the same fat loss principles as losing 100 pounds of excessive fat.

HOW DO WE LOSE FAT?

In order to lose fat you must create opposing circumstances to those that create fatness. Fatness is created by energy surplus, and to lose fat, you must create energy deficit. The only truth for fat loss is *energy deficit*. This is as sure as water is wet and fire is hot. Everything else is only clutter that confuses you.

> *The only truth for fat loss is ENERGY DEFICIT; this is as sure as the law of gravity! Everything else is only clutter that confuses you.*

In spite of that undeniable truth, many people justify their fatness and absence of fat loss with convenient, socially accepted excuses. "Tell me your secret," they plead, when they see someone who has lost fat. We are not talking about Houdini's magic tricks. There is no magic, there are no tricks or secrets. They should face the facts and create energy deficit by eating less and moving more.

Fat deposits on the body are like a gas tank on your car. If you refill less and drive more, the tank will empty. If you refill more and drive less, the tank will overspill. Fat on the body does not overspill, per se, but it does keep expanding.

COMMON MISUNDERSTANDING

By consuming less food and drinks and using more physical exercise, energy intake will decrease and energy expenditure will increase. That is true, but not necessarily enough for fat loss, because it does not automatically imply energy deficit. It does not work to just eat less if by eating "less" you are still eating too much. Similarly, it does not work to exercise "more" if you are still not exercising enough. Reduced nutrition and physical exercise are the best tools to create energy deficit, but those tools have to be used as long and as hard as necessary. Scratching a surface even with the best tools will not get the job done. Follow-through and commitment with the right tools will. For further explanation, see "Body lowers energy needs", page 84-86.

DON'T KILL THE MESSENGER

During a TV presentation of one of my books, I was talking about possible energy intake for fat loss diets. One lady from the live audience in the studio stood up and started complaining about how little food 1200 calories per day actually is. I told her then as I am telling you now: I did not design the human body and the rules of nature. I am just delivering the message.

I have a high regard for animals and nature. As humans we often arrogantly disregard their needs, wisdom and the lessons they offer us. When I have a dilemma, I find it eye-opening to resort to examples in nature for clarification. One such dilemma could be, "Are we designed to live from a high or low calorie intake?" or more abstractly, "Are we designed to survive in a luxury or restrictive environment?"

The answer is the latter in both cases. If our original design were for us to survive only from a high calorie intake and in luxurious life conditions, we would not have made it this far in our existence as a species. Only recently have we created an environment to provide access to plenty of food and conveniences. We are abusing this new luxury environment, satisfying cravings of our minds, not real needs of our bodies.

Look at the Serengeti (no, not the sunglasses, the national park in Tanzania). You don't even have to go that far and exotic, just look at your own backyard. Wild animals don't get luxury, but rather very limited resources for survival, and they do survive. They wait, work and fight hard for food, as we had to do throughout our history. Our bodies were also designed to live from a low calorie intake while performing hard physical labor. That is our original design, whether you like it or not. Our denial of it by "couch potato and buttered popcorn" behavior causes today's epidemic of fatness and obesity.

CUT IT OFF OR SUE SOMEONE

These days it is also considered normal to fantasize about a "magic fat loss pill", or better yet, to surgically suck out fat or even cut off a chunk of stomach, instead of just changing one's lifestyle. Figuratively speaking, I am not sure that I need to cut off my arm because it's picking my nose, or that I have to cut off my leg because it walks me in the wrong direction. Similarly, why would I have to sue a restaurant chain because I ate too much of their food and I am too fat?

My thoughts are the reason I pick my nose and walk in a wrong direction. It's not some restaurant chain deciding what and how much I eat and exercise, it's me. If I cannot control my thoughts now, why should I believe I will be able to control them any better missing my arm or leg, or having a law suit against some restaurant chain? Everything starts and ends with your mind. If you haven't dealt with your mind, no external circumstances alone will ever make you happy.

SURPLUS, BALANCE AND DEFICIT

Fatness and leanness come down to balance between consumed and used energy. To increase fat deposits you must consume more energy than your body needs (energy surplus). To maintain your current level of fat you must consume the same amount of energy that your body needs (energy balance). To lose fat you must consume less energy than your body needs (energy deficit). Fatness or absence of it is always and only a result of energy in and energy out, as a function of life's daily equation.

THE BEST TOOLS
FOR FAT LOSS

The best we can do to create an energy deficit, and therefore reduce fat deposits, are two things:

- Consume energy-reduced but, for health reasons, also well-balanced nutrition.
- Utilize physical activity, optimally aerobic exercise and resistance training.

A proper diet will provide the basic foundation for fat loss, namely, reduced energy intake. Aerobic exercise will burn plenty of energy and speed up the fat burning process. Resistance training will protect or even occasionally develop muscles during the fat loss process. Can a person lose fat by skipping one or more of these components? Yes, but the results might not be as satisfactory as when all these components are present properly.

FAT LOSS ONLY BY DIET

The most important component in losing fat is energy-reduced nutrition. Creating energy deficit only by reducing your nutrition will certainly make you lose fat. However, if you try to lose fat by dieting only, without adequate physical activity, the process is slower, less effective, and there is a bigger chance of undesirable muscle loss.

During fat loss it will be easier to stick with your diet if you exercise physically. Physical exercise will preoccupy your mind and fill up your daily schedule, so less time will be directed towards thinking about eating. When the body is physically active, somehow it makes more sense and feels easier to be a bit hungry.

If I diet for fat loss without exercise, it feels like I am losing both lean body mass and fat. That really can happen, but my feeling is exaggerated. It almost feels like I am rapidly disappearing. However, when I incorporate proper physical exercise there is a strong distinction between retaining lean body mass and removing excessive fat tissue. It feels like my lean body mass is a concrete surface (like a side walk) with a layer of dirt on the top, which is fat. Then when I lose fat by diet and exercise, it is like I am washing off dirt with a high-pressure hose, ending up with a solid and clean concrete surface.

If I diet for fat loss without physical exercise, it feels like there is only dirt, with no concrete underneath. As I wash the dirt off with a hose, no matter how much is washed away, I can never reach a solid, clean surface. It always feels like muddy sidewalk.

Maintaining muscles during fat loss is important for several reasons.

Aesthetics

No matter how much fat you lose, if there are no nicely shaped muscles, you will not be happy with the way your body looks. Muscles, not skin and bones, give nice shape and curve to our bodies.

Function

Muscles will give you more strength and power for daily life or sport activities.

Convenience

If you have more muscle your energy needs will be higher, meaning you can consume more energy and still lose fat. Muscle tissue requires more energy for its existence than fat tissue.

I believe aesthetics and function are good reasons for maintaining muscle mass. However, I am not so sure about convenience as a reason. Some will use this as an explanation for how it is easier to diet and lose fat with more muscle; that is, because you can eat more and, therefore, be less hungry. When I competed I was losing fat with an energy consumption of 3500 calories per day because of high muscle mass. Now with less muscle mass, I need to eat significantly less calories to realize the same dynamics of fat loss. Yet, in spite of the different amounts of calories I eat, I feel equally hungry during my fat loss now as I did then.

Regardless of relative muscle mass, when you want to lose fat you have to be hungry. Hunger is mostly generated by energy deficit, not by the sheer number of calories you consume. If the sheer number of calories, rather than energy deficit, were the major cause of hunger, an elephant would never be hungry because he eats so much food, that is, he has such a high calorie intake. On the other hand, a mouse would be hungry all the time because he cannot eat as much as an elephant can and his calorie intake is low.

FAT LOSS ONLY BY EXERCISE

Usually physical activity without proper diet will not be enough to lose fat, regardless of the amount or type of physical exercise. If you don't change your nutrition, you can lose fat by incorporating exercise if your current energy intake is at or very close to the maintenance level. Maintenance level means consumption of energy equals expenditure of energy. At that intake level, you maintain your current body weight. Then, by adding exercise, you will increase expenditure of a few hundred calories per day, and cause fat loss due to newly created energy deficit. Even if that happens, and that happens rarely, it will not last long enough to cause significant or complete fat loss. Additionally, if you start with physical activity, but also increase food intake and consume more calories than before, physical activity will not result in losing fat. Then, you might even get fatter.

Train in vain

Do remember this: *you cannot generate enough physical activity to burn the excessive energy that can be easily consumed in one oversized meal.*

After a big meal, people will often say that they have to go to the gym to burn it off. That is a huge misconception. You can spend hours in vain at the gym working out hard and still not burn even half of the calories from one oversized meal. If you are on a fat loss program and have consumed more than your planned amount of food in one meal, do not trouble yourself much by specially going to the gym to burn it off. Follow your usual routine and if your food craving is still high, I would suggest you take a whole day off, have more food, relax and start fresh tomorrow.

For example, when I take a day off and let myself go, I easily consume 15,000 calories that day. Consider what it takes to burn this many calories. When I competed and did very hard leg workouts (leg workouts usually expend the most energy), I was expending about 1200-1500 calories each 90-minute training. Therefore, to burn off those easily consumed 15,000 calories, I would have to do about 10 intense 90-minute leg workouts in the same day, which is practically impossible. Moreover, a typical gym member does not spend 1200-1500 calories per workout, but usually less than 500.

Now do yourself a favor and don't get stuck on my numbers, thinking, "Oh, I can't eat that much", or "Oh, I can't train that much, so this example doesn't apply to me." Receive the message, regardless of unimportant details like the size of the body, level of gluttony or intensity of the workout. The same goes for all other examples I use in the book.

The message you should receive from this example is that there is almost no point in trying to lose fat just by physical exercise if you do not diet properly. The vast majority of people do not understand that. Often they start exercising in the gym thinking exercise alone will do it. It will not.

Whenever I tried to lose fat only by exercise and without diet, I did not reach my fat loss goal, but even worse, I lost the desire to keep exercising. It felt to me like there was no point in exercising since I wasn't seeing results, or at least not fast enough. On the other hand, when I exercise along with a proper diet, I am more tired and hungry because of the reduced nutritional intake, but the obvious progress towards my fat loss goal improves my motivation for exercise and fat loss exponentially. Of course, physical exercise has a positive effect on your body in general, even if you do not lose fat.

Without a doubt, if you are serious about fat loss, the best you can do is apply a suitable nutritional and exercise program. One without the other is just not good enough if the best is what you are after.

BEFORE		AFTER

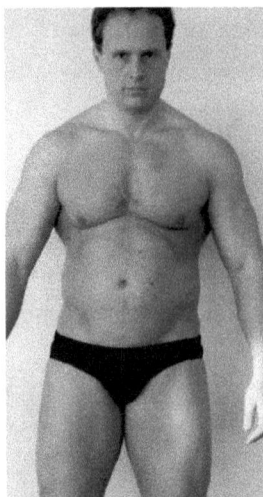 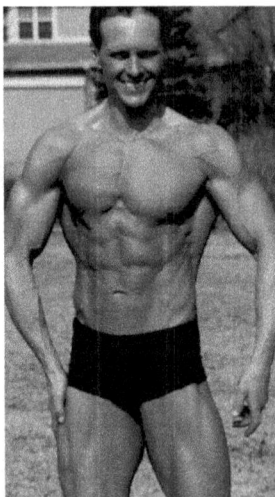

1/21/2002	*3 MONTHS*	4/21/2002
250 lbs	*LATER*	190 lbs
24% body fat		3.1% body fat

CHAPTER THREE

Chapter Three confronts common thinking that fast food restaurants are concentrated sources of evil, that they are the reason for today's epidemic of obesity, and should be lynched, or at least sued and robbed of their money. This chapter certifies that, contrary to fat loss myths, you can actually eat wherever and whatever you wish and still lose fat. You are also granted asylum from "must-join-gym" mentality.

FATNESS AND ITS USUAL SUSPECTS

Let's address this mangy question. "Why do we have more fat people now than 100 years ago?" I don't know for sure, though I mostly agree with common opinion, that more technology requires less mandatory physical effort both at work and at home. These days we usually have to choose to do physical work (exercise) if we want to be physically active, and this was not so only 100 years ago. Back then, manual labor was more a mandatory part of life for most people. We now use less and consume more energy than before, resulting in an energy surplus which leads to increased fatness.

If we are already physically less active, why do we consume more energy? One hundred years ago, we had only a "few" kinds of meats, fruits and vegetables available, and we had to work hard to obtain and prepare them. These days, a vast variety of different foods with countless delicious tastes are available almost all the time for much less effort. As a result, people are tempted more often, and the objects of their temptations are more accessible. The outcome is the epidemic of fatness. Some sources say that today, on average, we weigh about 25 pounds more than only 40 years ago.

> **Don't blame others for your fatness. What you eat for your fit or fat figure is your choice.**

Knowing these facts and considering human nature, it is absolutely understandable and normal that we are fatter these days than before. Would it also be normal to expect that after a day of work and stress, when we can finally relax a bit, that we would choose to invest even more effort into non-mandatory physical work (that is, exercise) and restrain ourselves from foods we like? Of course not, even though it would be better for us to do so.

FINDING SOMEONE TO BLAME

How do we stop this negative trend of obesity, and who is to blame? We stop it by balancing our lives better and choosing wisely. If we need to blame someone, we blame ourselves for past wrong choices. I am absolutely against blaming fast food restaurants or other popular targets. They are just convenient scapegoats, with enough money to become targets of laughable lawsuits.

Blaming fast food restaurants for your fatness or poor food choices is equally as inappropriate as blaming grocery stores for selling chocolate, ice-cream, or butter. This is absurd thinking! The physical fitness of customers is not their responsibility. In fact, restaurants and stores do not and should not have any responsibility in the matter, unless they sell tainted or falsely-advertised products. What food you eat for your fit or fat figure is your choice and exclusively your responsibility.

LOSE FAT
IN FAST FOOD PLACES DAILY

I guarantee, you can successfully lose fat and not jeopardize your health by eating daily in any popular fast food restaurant. Forget about those manipulative, frustrated and biased movies portraying them as "monsters of modern civilization". My clients and I have lost fat by eating in fast food restaurants many times. What matters is what, and how much, you consume from their menus. You do not have to super-size it! Why would you?

Moreover, people are eager to point the finger at fast food places but don't complain about fancy restaurants (except maybe their prices). Do you think you cannot over-eat in five-star restaurants, consume too much fat, choke on desserts, get sick, clog your arteries, and so forth? Yes you can. At least in fast food restaurants you can do it for less money.

I am not saying you should camp out in fast food restaurants. I am saying that fast food restaurants are all over the place, and considering the busy life style of many, it is almost impossible to avoid them. They play an important role, making affordable food available easily and quickly. You can benefit from these advantages, even during your fat loss program.

The bottom line is we should all be grateful for the vast variety of foods that are available nearly all the time, and for the fact that we don't have to do as much physical labor as before. What is there to complain about? If something generally good is available to you, it is preposterous to abuse it and blame it later. That would be like blaming the car when a drunk driver causes a collision. Your abuse of something good does not turn the original good nature of it into something bad. As my father, Josip, likes to say, "If you just don't do what hurts you, you'll be fine".

> *Eating healthy is related to eating for fat loss like the English language is related to Spanish.*

EAT WHATEVER YOU WANT

You can eat any kind of food, and still lose fat and body weight. You can even eat fast food, ice cream, chocolate, pizza, candy, processed food, packaged food, and other popular so-called "evils," and still lose fat. How is this possible? I will repeat: it is not important what you eat, but instead how much you eat. *Energy deficit is the only truth for fat loss.* Everything else is only clutter that confuses you. This is the undeniable fact. If you forget everything else from this book, remember this.

BUT I EAT HEALTHY

People often complain that they eat healthy but cannot lose fat. Of course they can't. They eat too much, healthy or not. Eating healthy is related to eating for fat loss like the English language is related to Spanish. They do have things in common, but not enough to establish successful communication.

Furthermore, what does it mean to eat healthy? For some people eating healthy means eating vegetables and skipping chocolate; for others, it means something

> *You can eat the "healthiest" food, but if you eat too much, you will still get fat. Types of food don't cause fatness – lack of temperance does.*

different. Regardless, you can choose the "healthiest" food known to mankind, but if you eat too much of it, you will still get fat, and therefore not be eating healthy! Eating a moderate amount of energy is one of the most important components of genuinely healthy eating.

Back to our previously listed so-called "evil" foods like fast food, pizza and candy. Can you eat moderate amounts of energy if you eat such foods? Yes you can, but you usually have to stop eating much sooner than you would like to because these foods taste so good. That's where discipline must kick in. Besides tasting so good, these foods usually have more energy than equal amounts of other foods considered diet-friendly and "good". For instance 3 ounces of chocolate contains about 500 calories, while 3 ounces of tomato contains less than 20 calories. Therefore, you have to eat approximately 0.1 ounces of chocolate to consume the same amount of energy as from 3 ounces of tomato. Types of food are not to be blamed for fatness and unsuccessful fat loss. Our lack of temperance is to be blamed.

> **Balance food in the way that fits you the best, but stay in energy deficit.**

I want to repeat what I said in the beginning. You absolutely should eat well balanced and healthy nutrition. What kind of nutrition is well balanced and healthy for your individual needs, is a decision you will have to make on your own or in cooperation with your physician and nutritionist. This book is not designed to provide such advice. Once you have chosen the type of nutrition, this book will teach you how to adapt it to lose excessive body fat. By losing excessive body fat you should improve your health and well-being.

AMOUNT VS. TASTE

When you go on a fat loss diet, you have to make a choice about what kind of food to include in your daily menu. The right choice should be an individually suitable combination of both low-energy low-taste food, and high-energy high-flavored food. If you decide to go for better tasting food, you will have to consume less of it because such foods usually release much more energy. Of course, if you can find low-energy and high-flavor food, go for it.

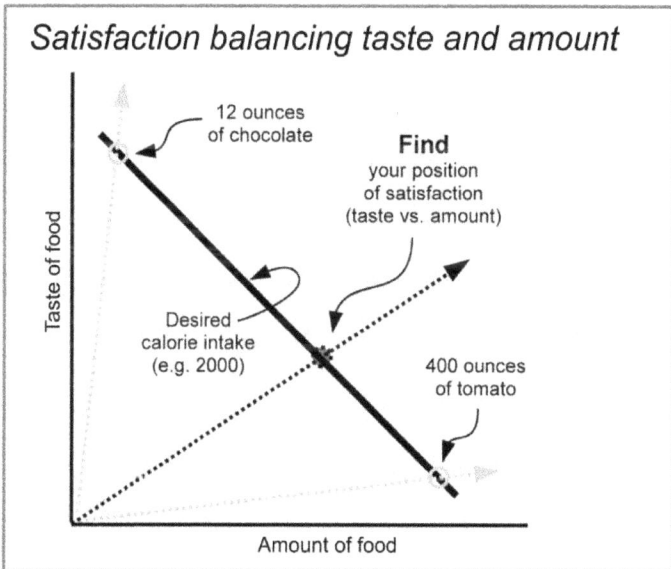

Satisfaction balancing taste and amount

12 ounces of chocolate

Find your position of satisfaction (taste vs. amount)

Taste of food

Desired calorie intake (e.g. 2000)

400 ounces of tomato

Amount of food

Balance your food choices the way that satisfies you the best, but remain within an energy deficit. This is how and why you can eat whatever you want and lose fat.

> *Control your mind, and it will lead your body to successful fat loss.*

When I diet, I consume foods with less energy and stay away from tasty foods. I have an old fashioned approach, "The harder the better. If it tastes good it is not good for my fat loss". Other than my days off, my menus mostly contain the same five to seven foods from day one until the end, typically two to four months later. By eating this way, I feel I achieve the best balance between my invested effort and fat loss reward.

> *Don't adapt yourself to fit the diet – adapt the diet to fit you. Diet the way you are. Lose fat by embracing your own strengths, weaknesses and desires.*

Remember, during fat loss your mind is usually the weakest link. Control your mind and it will lead your body in the right direction.

For safe and efficient fat loss, satisfy your mind with preferred choices of food within reason, but stay inside your appropriate number of calories and other required nutrients. Design your diet completely from scratch, or combine aspects of two or more diets together, and create your own original approach. Do not adapt yourself to fit a particular diet, adapt the diet to fit your particular needs. Diet the way you are.

This fact, that you can eat whatever you want to in your own way, flies in the face of common beliefs and boldly encourages you not to fearfully follow someone else's diet and have to deal with parts that don't suit you. It empowers you to courageously embrace your own strengths, weaknesses and desires, and create your own fat loss matrix of success.

THE BODY KNOWS NUTRITION

Even if we are not conscious of it, the healthy body automatically knows what nutrition it needs, and will lead us in the right direction. When nutrients are required the body will create hunger and cravings for particular foods, and those foods will be consumed. Then the body will use what is available to satisfy its needs. When I say craving for a particular food, I refer to physical cravings. I do not mean an emotional craving for an additional slice of apple pie after a hefty meal, nor a craving for an oversized carton of buttered popcorn before a movie. Physical cravings enable you to survive; emotional cravings make you fat.

We learned a lot about food and nutrition only very recently in our history. How did we survive all those thousands of years before we obtained our current knowledge? Did cave men know about the biochemistry of nutrition? Do animals know anything about it? I don't think they consciously do, but their bodies definitely know what they need and where to get it.

BEAR WITH A HORMONAL IMBALANCE
EATING CHOCOLATE

Consider a simple example. A bear can eat almost anything, yet from all those choices (without knowing consciously) he picks the right ones. Even when he doesn't pick the right ones, his body compensates. The best proof is the fact that he is alive and healthy. Furthermore, before winter he gets fat by eating plenty of "healthy" food. He eats lots of "vegetables" and he does not eat chocolate or fast food. Then, after getting fat on his healthy nutrition, he goes to hibernate. In the spring, he is lean again, because he did not eat much during the winter.

> *The bear did not make any drama. He just reduced energy intake, created energy deficit, and lost fat.*

Did he have a hormonal imbalance that kept him from losing fat? No, but even if he had, he would still lose fat! Did he have to eat more during winter in order to speed up his metabolism to burn fat? No, he did not! He did not create any drama or mystery about such a simple and natural thing as fat loss. He reduced energy intake, created an energy deficit, and lost fat.

BEARS AND CAVE MEN
KNOW THEIR STUFF

I am not suggesting we should live and eat like cave men or bears. I am suggesting that our body still "knows" much better than our science how to eat, exercise and survive. You should use its' hints with properly measured attitude. I also suggest you gather as much current knowledge as you can, but be very selective and careful in applying it. Our knowledge is too often abused for commercial purposes. So called "scientific information" is used to disguise heartless, money-making schemes as fairy-tales, suggesting that if you buy a particular product, you will lose fat. I suggest you put logic and laws of nature ahead of such tempting, wolf-in-sheep's-clothing commercial promises. And when you are not sure about your logic or your own understanding of the laws of nature, simply look back at nature logically and you will have your answers. Somehow bears and cave men knew what they were doing.

> *The body knows how to eat, exercise and survive much better than science does.*

MUST I GO
TO A FITNESS CENTER?

If you have decided to go to a fitness center, you have made a great decision and have given yourself the opportunity to utilize the best exercise tools for successful fat loss. In a contemporary fitness center you will have a variety of cardio machines, as well as resistance training machines. Fitness centers commonly offer other valuable services such as assistance from professional trainers, classes, a swimming pool and so on. However, getting into shape doesn't necessarily require a wide variety of equipment and services. In the beginning, start with a simple but effective program, and then expand your program if new needs arise.

> *A burning desire and strong discipline are the best fat loss partners.*

Using a fitness center will be a great help and drastically increase your chances of success. But fat does not evaporate just because you paid for a membership or training sessions. You have to work smart and hard to burn it off. A person with a burning desire and strong discipline will be more successful in burning fat just by walking a dog, than a person without desire and discipline in the best fitness center and with the best trainer. Fitness centers are not a guarantee of fat loss success. Your attitude is the strongest guarantee of your success.

For those of you who are already gym members, here is some advice. When you don't feel like going to the gym, go anyway with the intention of completing an easy workout. You will either be glad you at least followed through with an easy workout, or more likely, since you are already there, little by little you will end up having completed a pretty good workout. However, if you don't feel like going to the gym because you are sick, hurt or have some other justified reason, then don't go until you are ready again.

WALK THE DOG INSTEAD

A good fitness center is the best place to find all the exercise equipment needed for burning fat. However, if you are opposed to the idea of going to a fitness center, or getting involved in other kinds of structured exercising, you still can lose fat very successfully.

Any kind of physical work will increase energy expenditure and, therefore, is a great aid in fat loss. Burned energy is burned energy, regardless of whether it comes from scientifically planned sports conditioning, or random manual labor in your back yard.

> *Sports competition or cleaning the house – burned energy is burned energy.*

You can walk the dog, use stairs instead of the elevator, go for a bike ride, clean up the house, or do just about anything else that requires physical effort and is safe at the same time. By doing any of these, you will burn more energy as compared to a sedentary lifestyle. However, these activities are not a substitute for the benefits of proper resistance training. They may burn more calories, but they cannot precisely train each muscle group as resistance training can.

How long to do physical exercise or work depends on your physical condition and health. Do not overly stress the body. Increase the intensity and duration of physical effort gradually. Keep that in mind and be physically active as often and as long as realistically possible. The bottom line is to be physically active. If you are sitting on a couch and watching TV, your body may burn about 50-100 calories per hour. However, if you instead clean your house, during that time your body may be spending about 200-300 calories per hour.

USE DYNAMIC
FULL BODY MOVEMENTS

When choosing activities to increase energy expenditure it is better to actively involve more and bigger muscle groups. Any dynamic exercise or work that requires all or most of your body to move will do just fine. Choose something that will noticeably increase your heart rate, breathing rhythm and perspiration, but do not exaggerate the intensity of it (see "Aerobic physical activities", page 214-218).

For example, if you physically exercise three hours, but only use your forearms while the rest of your body is sitting and relaxing, you will not burn enough energy to notice any contribution to your fat loss. Forearms are a very small muscle group and they will get tired, but overall your body will still be fresh and rested. In contrast, if you do squats and use comparatively large muscle groups like your legs and back, you will burn more energy in just a "few minutes" and better help your fat loss. Similarly, do not just complete hours of passive stretching while watching TV, try something more vigorous. For instance, watch TV while walking on a treadmill or riding a stationary bike.

To achieve fat loss, in addition to your diet, (1) it is best to use well-structured resistance training and aerobic exercise in a contemporary fitness center; (2) it is good enough to use any kind of safe and energy demanding physical effort (exercise or work); but (3) it is not good to be physically passive and live a sedentary life, in consideration of not only your fat loss, but also the health, function and aesthetics of your body.

CHAPTER FOUR

In this chapter you are going to find out what really happens during a sound fat loss program. How many pounds can you lose per week? How much might your body weight fluctuate during your fat loss? What about plateaus and spot fat reduction? What does it take to maintain your new, lean body condition? Chapter Four answers these questions based on numerous successes and failures I had as an athlete, trainer, author and regular guy that just wants to lose fat.

VELOCITY OF FAT LOSS

There is no such thing as an exact and universal number of pounds a person should lose weekly during fat loss. The number depends on many factors, like body size, gender, specifics of the body, how much total fat you want to lose, and so on. Therefore, when certain values are suggested take them only as approximate guidelines.

Having said this, my usual fat loss recommendation is half a pound to two pounds per week. In cases of individuals with very small or large body sizes, these values can be lower or higher, respectively. Bodies are like car engines. A smaller engine will generally use less gas (energy) than a bigger engine. Half a pound to two pounds of fat loss per week should not demand too much effort and, at the same time, it should be fairly safe for lean body mass (muscle tissue). Half a pound to two pounds per week may sound like a small amount, but if you multiply it by 52 weeks, you end up losing 26 to 104 pounds of fat per year.

When I suggest a half to two pounds per week, consider it as an average value of fat loss during a longer period of time (a few weeks, or longer), not as an exact value you have to achieve every single week. Even if you try, you cannot be that precise. Numbers will change from one week to the next even if you are basically on the exact same fat loss plan. On average, though, you can be in the ballpark.

LOSE IT EVEN FASTER

In cases of substantial fatness, for motivational reasons, you can create a program for even faster fat loss. When you see obvious signs of fat loss, motivation becomes stronger, and chances of giving up are decreased. Obvious signs of success are excellent motivators for further efforts.

As an example, imagine that you have 150 pounds of excess fat. By losing only one pound of fat per week, you will have reached your fat loss goal in 150 weeks (almost three years). Over such a long period of time, you are very likely to give up. On the other hand, if you start losing four pounds per week, the numbers change drastically. 150 pounds of excessive fat will be eliminated not in three years, but in less than nine months, which will help you maintain the required level of motivation.

The four pounds per week example is exaggerated. Not many people have the body size and capacity to maintain such an intensive fat loss for a prolonged period of time. Even if they do in the beginning, such a rate could slow down in later stages of fat loss. Understand and accept this principle, but adjust the numbers to your needs and capacity. Never push yourself beyond safe and acceptable limits.

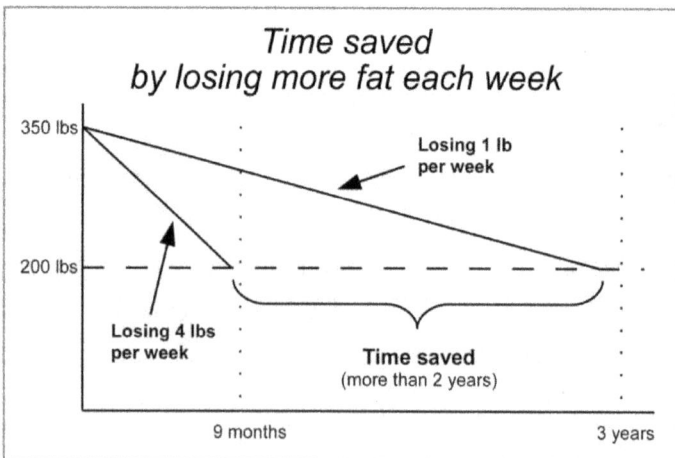

Time saved by losing more fat each week

350 lbs

Losing 1 lb per week

200 lbs

Losing 4 lbs per week

Time saved (more than 2 years)

9 months   3 years

For example, for one of my books, I once tested how much body weight reduction I could achieve during a one month period without overly exhausting myself. During that month I lost 25.3 pounds (11.5 kg) which is about 5.9 pounds per week, or 0.84 pounds per day. On the other hand, during one competition conditioning period, lasting about three months, my weight loss was slower, resulting in a reduction of about 3.5 pounds per week, or a half pound per day. In the latter case, the process was noticeably slower due to the extended duration of fat loss. Using running as an example, your maximum running speed will be higher during a 100-meter race, than during a one-mile race.

HOW TO SPEED UP FAT LOSS

If you want to speed up fat loss, the process conceptually stays the same; it is just applied more aggressively. Simply put, you have to generate more hunger and create a larger energy deficit. Consume less energy and increase the amount of exercise.

Keep in mind that very fat people with a high body weight will be limited in their capacity to perform physically. For them even slow walking can be very demanding and an efficient form of exercise. Therefore, proper adjustments in choice and execution of exercise have to be made for each person, and, to be on the safe side, medical supervision is a must.

It is believed that if you lose a very large amount of fat too quickly, then your skin will not have enough time to adapt to the new smaller volume of the body, and it will "hang loose". I am not sure if that is correct. I am more inclined to think that skin has difficulty adapting if it loses its elasticity due to age or other factors like stretch marks or scarring. If that is the case, then regardless of how slow or fast you lose fat, your skin will still sag.

WEIGHT LOSS CURVES

When you start losing fat, body weight reduction will exhibit different dynamics of change.

INITIAL
QUANTUM WEIGHT DROP

At the very beginning, it is realistic to expect almost an instant and significant weight loss. That happens when a sudden switch from higher energy nutrition to lower energy nutrition is applied. In extreme cases a person can lose 10 or more pounds in the first three to five days. How much the person is going to lose depends on body size, change in nutrition, level of physical activity and other factors. This initial quantum weight drop during the first three to five days should not be factored into the calculation of how many pounds of body weight you can lose during a week of your fat loss dieting.

A sudden initial quantum weight drop is a normal occurrence caused by emptying the digestive system and by water release. It does not represent sudden fat loss by any means. In the later stages, weight loss becomes much slower, and if done correctly, it will represent real fat loss.

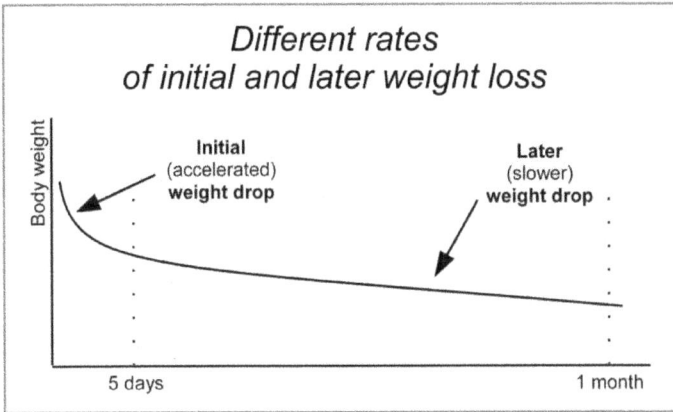

Different rates of initial and later weight loss

LATER
STEP-LIKE WEIGHT DROP

During the later stages of your fat loss program, recognizable fat loss is not as obvious on a daily basis. Even when constantly in the state of energy deficit, weight loss will happen in a step-like, descending curve. Such a curve will show short periods of maintaining the same body weight (or even slight weight increases), followed by "overnight" sudden drops in body weight. However, these drops are not nearly as big as the initial quantum weight drop. This is normal and such cycles will keep happening throughout the period of fat loss. Even when you have completed your fat loss program and want to maintain the same, lower body weight, your weight will not be identical every day, though it will stay very close to the desired number.

These sudden step-like drops in body weight will not happen in consistent time intervals and they will not always have the same value in pounds, even if you stay with the same fat loss program. One interval may last four days and you may lose one pound, while another may last only two days and you may lose two pounds. Typically the stricter your diet, especially during the beginning stage of your fat loss, the more likely you will have greater drops of body weight.

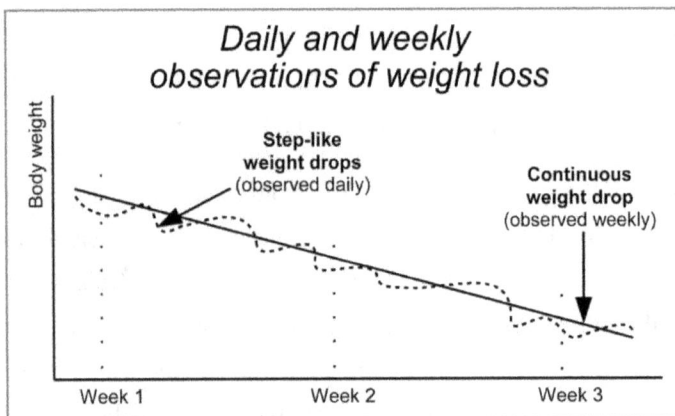

Daily and weekly observations of weight loss

Such step-like body weight fluctuations, if observed on a daily basis, could even show frequent ups and downs from one day to the next. However, if weight fluctuations are observed on a weekly or better yet monthly basis, results should descend continuously.

Even though you may not see progress by checking your body weight daily, do not let that bother you. If you are on a proper program, you are still losing fat. If not noticing daily weight loss bothers you, check your weight only once or twice a week. If you do not drop body weight within a week or longer, then you are consuming too much energy and require a more strict fat loss program. Every new week of your fat loss you should weigh a bit less than the previous week, and certainly less than the weeks before that.

Conversely, when you gain fat, your increase in body weight happens in the same way, but in the opposite direction, by a step-like ascending curve instead of a descending curve. That means, if observed on a daily basis, body weight could show the same values over a few days, or even occasional drops, but over a longer period, results will have ascending tendencies.

KEEP LOSING,
STOP LOSING, KEEP LOSING

When losing fat, if there is plenty of fat to lose and no deadline pressure, do not strive necessarily for constant fat (weight) loss, as observed on a weekly or monthly basis. Sometimes it is a good idea to lose some fat–for example, 10 pounds–and then keep the body weight at the same level for a while. Then, one month later, you could decide to continue progress towards your final goal and lose another five pounds. Then hold your weight right there for a few weeks. Each period of losing fat does not have to be equally intensive. Continue this pattern until you reach your goal.

Keep alternating periods of energy deficit for fat loss, with periods of energy balance for maintenance of the same body weight, but do not go into extended periods of energy surplus.

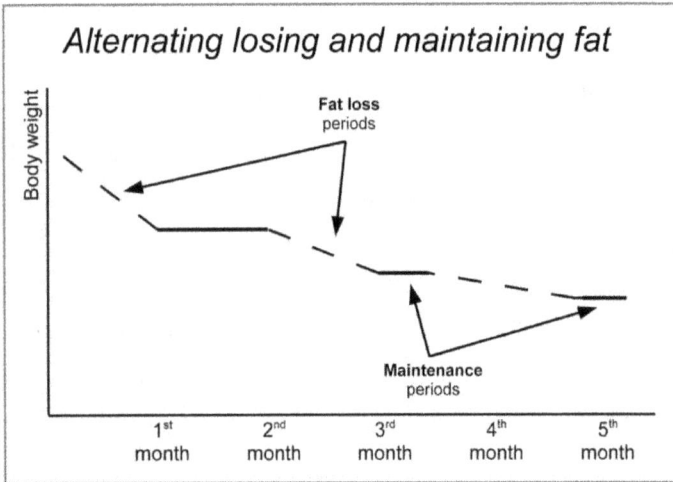

One of the greatest advantages you can give yourself during fat loss is not to rush it. Take your time. However, keep progressing towards your goal. I think periods of maintaining the same body weight during an ongoing fat loss process should not last longer than a month, because they could interrupt your fat loss rhythm.

AIMING FOR EXACT
BODY WEIGHT

If your goal is to have a certain body weight, rather than just navigate your fat loss according to how you look and feel, you must understand that when you are done losing fat, you need to increase your food intake a bit and exercise differently, otherwise you will keep losing fat. At that time, your body could retain more fluid and food, and your body weight could increase a bit.

If you are dropping your body weight, for instance, from 150 pounds and wish to have a stable, daily body weight of 120 pounds, ideally you should aim for reaching 115 pounds at the end of your fat loss program (as the lowest recorded body weight). If you stop when you reach 120 pounds, then after you change your nutrition and exercise, there is a chance you will end up a few pounds heavier than your desired daily weight (e.g. 125 pounds).

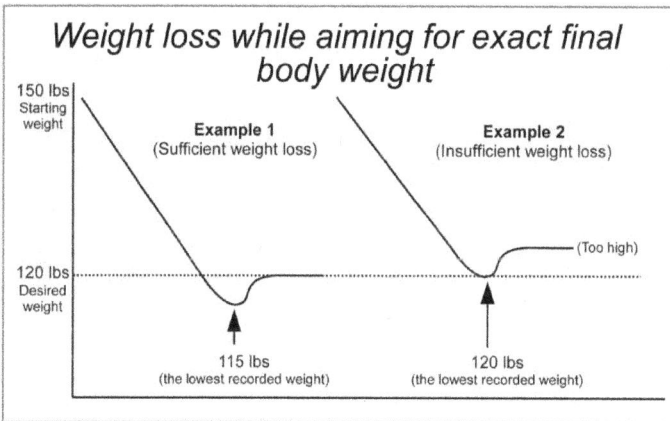

Weight loss while aiming for exact final body weight

150 lbs
Starting weight

Example 1
(Sufficient weight loss)

Example 2
(Insufficient weight loss)

(Too high)

120 lbs
Desired weight

115 lbs
(the lowest recorded weight)

120 lbs
(the lowest recorded weight)

This is especially the case if you measure your body weight every morning on an empty stomach after using the bathroom. That measure of body weight is generally a bit lower than your "normal" daily body weight measured in the middle of the day after food and drink consumption.

BODY LOWERS ENERGY NEEDS

When you reduce your energy intake, your body will lower its energy needs to a certain extent to try to match the lower intake. The body wants to establish balance between energy in and energy out. For example, if you were successfully losing fat consuming 2000 calories per day at the beginning of your fat loss, after a couple of weeks or a month, your body could decrease its energy needs, and you could stop losing fat at that same 2000 calorie per day energy intake level. When your progress stops (or slows down), you have to create (or increase) energy deficit again by either reducing energy intake, or by increasing energy expenditure. You can also do both, eat less and move more.

How long it will take before you stop losing fat depends on the degree of energy deficit that was created with your initial daily energy intake. Make no mistake, this will not go on indefinitely. The body can reduce its energy needs only so much. After a certain point, you will keep losing fat even if you never decrease your energy intake again.

Regardless of how physically active or inactive you may be, the body needs a substantial amount of energy just for basic life functions, and that energy will be used as long as you are alive. In many cases for the average physically active individual, the body will need more energy for basic life functions than for all other daily activities together.

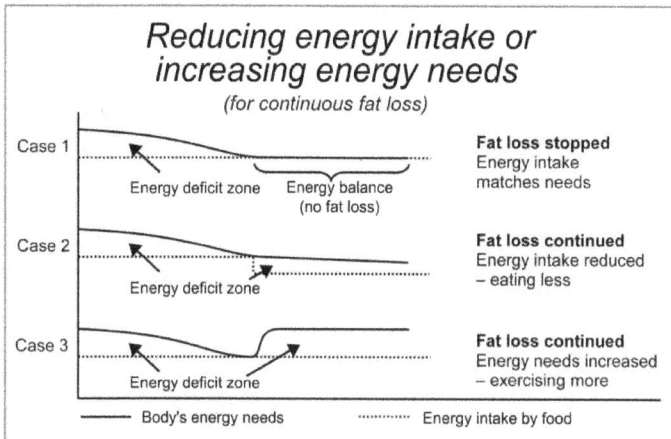

Here is an example of a reduction in energy intake during a fat loss program due to the body's reduced energy needs. My basal metabolic rate (BMR) used to be 3570 calories per day. That was the amount of energy I needed only for my body to function while awake and at rest. When we add to this trainings and daily activities, I needed about 6000 calories or more to maintain my body weight.

With an assumed energy requirement of 6000 calories per day, I started my fat loss diet at 4500 calories per day. That energy intake level provided good fat loss for a while. After approximately 2-3 weeks, I needed to further reduce my energy intake to 3500 calories. Finally, to continue with my target rate of fat loss, I had to reduce my energy intake as low as 2500 calories per day. Even if I did not reduce my energy intake all the way to 2500 calories per day, my body would still burn fat with a bit higher energy intake, but wouldn't have lost fat as fast as I needed in order to meet my deadline.

One of the reasons for the body's reduced energy needs is due to weight loss itself. A body that weighs less will need less energy to live, move and work.

FAT LOSS PLATEAUS,
NO SUCH THING

While losing fat, plateaus will not happen as long as you are in energy deficit. If your body reduces its energy needs and you stop losing fat, simply consume less energy and the problem will be solved. You will stop losing fat if you eat too much, but that is not a plateau in the real sense of the word.

To illustrate what a real plateau is, consider the process of developing muscle. When developing muscle, even if you do everything to the best of current knowledge and exert your highest reasonable effort, the result is still not guaranteed. The muscle gain process is slow, limited and packed with plateaus. Such cases can be considered plateaus because they will happen in spite of your efforts. On the other hand, when it comes to fat loss, even if you now have 50% body fat, you can drop your fat percentage under 10%

if you keep losing fat the right way and over a long enough period of time.

If you consciously decide to keep your body weight at a certain level before you continue further fat loss, that is not a plateau (as explained in "Keep losing, stop losing, keep losing"). Similarly, a plateau is not a short maintenance period of a certain body weight during a step-like weight drop that happens in the later stages of the diet (as explained in "Later step-like weight drops").

SPOT FAT REDUCTION, WISHFUL THINKING

We often hear that we can achieve fat reduction on only one body part. It is impossible to reduce fat from only one chosen part of the body, while the other parts stay "untouched". Think about fat deposits on the body as the gas tank in your car. You cannot empty only the front left corner of that tank, because the gas will equally empty from all parts of the tank. The same applies for fat reduction in the body.

SIX PACK
BY DIET, NOT BY SIT UPS

Many people think if they exercise a fatter body part more, they will increase fat reduction from that body part. They will not. Working muscles do not "suck out" energy only from fat in their close proximity. It is "sucked out" from all over the body. The most common body parts under such misconception are the stomach (six pack), waist and lower back area, buttocks, thighs and backs of the upper arms.

For instance, to burn fat from your stomach and show your six pack, it is not necessary to drastically increase your amount of abdominal muscle exercises. You simply have to start with overall fat loss. The problem is the quantity of fat that covers them up, rather than your muscle mass, shape or firmness. People achieve a "six pack" stomach by losing fat, sometimes even without training abdominal muscles at all.

SEXY ABS – POSSESSION OF ALL, NOT PRIVILEGE OF FEW

We all have six pack muscles underneath our skin, because what gives them their six pack shape is their specific structure. That is simply an anatomical fact of our species, not a privilege of a few, select individuals. However, some people do have more and some less developed six pack muscles. Regardless, no matter how developed they are, they will not be obvious if the layer of fat and skin on top of them is too thick. That is the main reason why bodybuilders have to reduce their body fat to the minimum level before a show (that process is referred to as "definition"). They have big muscles, but still must "thin their skin" so they can better reveal their six pack and other muscles. Therefore to tone, firm and define your body for everyday life, or a bodybuilding show, you must lose excessive fat.

Think about it like this. If a three-inch thick comforter covers your mattress, you will see only its basic rectangular

> *Doing sit-ups won't show your six pack – energy deficit will.*

shape. However, if the same mattress is covered only by a thin silk sheet, you will see its basic shape and also the fine details of its texture. The same principle applies to all body parts, so forget about spot fat reduction, and apply overall fat loss.

BOGEYMAN

Some body parts may exhibit different dynamics of losing fat. The body part that will appear to lose fat first (that is, become obviously leaner) could be a bit different for each body. Regardless, you cannot change the natural order of fat loss. It is important to know that excessive fat deposits can be removed from any body part if you lose fat correctly and long enough. Eventually you will burn off all excess.

Women, for example, often start fat loss to trim fat from their stomach, hips and thighs (fatter parts), while hoping not to lose any fat from the chest and upper body (leaner parts). This scenario usually plays out completely differently. Expect that fat deposits will be reduced more obviously first from leaner body parts, while the fattest parts will initially appear like they are staying the same.

For this reason, many will panic and stop their fat loss program because in the beginning it seems that the lean areas get even leaner, and the fat areas stay the same. Don't be afraid of this Bogeyman; stopping is a mistake. You should continue losing fat because the process will "turn" towards the fatter body parts, and they will become obviously leaner.

These explanations are simplified, but the message is this. If a person keeps losing fat correctly and long enough, excessive fat will be removed from all body parts regardless of which one appeared to lose fat first or the most. For example, pinch the skin on the leanest part of your body right now. That is how thin (and likely even thinner) the skin on the fattest parts of your body can become when you are done losing fat. Keep in mind, energy deficit is an amazingly powerful (and the only genuine) tool for fat loss. If applied long enough it will burn off all excess fat.

$$$

One of the reasons why leaner body parts appear to lose fat sooner and faster than fatter body parts could be due to the smaller amount of fat. Think about it as a stack of money. If you have 100 bills, take a few out, and you will hardly notice the difference. But if you have only five bills and take a few out, the difference is noticeable.

The same principle is true with gaining fat. Accumulation of fat is going to be the most obvious in the beginning when the body is lean. At that time, every new pound of fat is very obvious. Later on, as the body gets fatter and fatter, every new pound is less and less obvious by itself, but it undeniably adds up eventually to obesity. That could be the reason why some individuals accumulate so much fat. Many even wonder how they let themselves get to that point. I think, after the first obvious awareness of getting fat occurs, and nothing is done about it, the rest sneaks in gradually over time.

COSMETIC SURGERY, NO BUT YES

As I have discussed previously, it is impossible through exercise and nutrition to keep fat on some body parts and remove it from others. Clearly, you should not train one body part more and expect such changes as they will not happen. That kind of partial, spot fat reduction is possible only by surgical intervention. I am against such an approach mostly for these two reasons.

First, results from cosmetic surgery will never be as natural and complete, nor even come close to results of fat loss accomplished by diet and exercise. Also, the chance of getting uneven results increases as the amount of removed fat from individual areas increases.

Second, cutting fat out removes the symptom, not the cause. The excessive fat will come back on the same or another part of your body if you do not change your lifestyle. And if you do change your lifestyle, why not take care of the problem the right way, without surgery? Fatness is not like cancer, there is no need for complicated and expensive methods to remove it.

I do support cosmetic surgeries in order to obtain results you might want that cannot be achieved naturally. However, if anything can or should be achieved naturally and by a conventional method, it is fat loss. Simply cut down on your food intake, and you will lose fat and save money. That said, in some cases of extreme fat reduction cosmetic surgery can help reduce excessive skin that does not successfully adjust to a new, smaller volume of body.

IT'S NOT FAT

Despite dubious messages to the contrary, any weight gain or weight loss that happens suddenly–for example, a few pounds in a few hours or even a few days–is not related to a change in the amount of fat deposits in the body. Fat gain and fat loss are fairly slow processes. However, body weight can change rapidly due to food or water retention or release.

To illustrate this point, consider that one pound of body fat contains about 3500 calories. Average daily energy needs for women are considered to be about 1700 calories. Therefore, to lose only one pound of fat, an average woman would have to eat and drink zero calories (that is, basically, she should not eat or drink) for two days while still performing her usual schedule. Along this same line of thinking, to lose 10 pounds of fat the same woman would have to maintain her normal schedule for 20 days without consuming any calories. That would put her into an energy deficit of the almost 35,000 calories required to lose about 10 pounds of fat.

While this scenario is obviously exaggerated and unrealistic, it makes the important point that fat gain and fat loss require significant time. Changes like that cannot happen overnight, or even over a couple of days. You did not get fat overnight, nor will you get lean overnight. The good news is you can lose fat in a shorter time than it took you to gain it. The bad news is you gained fat by careless and effortless behavior, but to lose it, you will have to care about it and invest considerable effort. Remember, sudden changes in body weight happen due to food or water retention or release, not fat gain or loss. If you're being told otherwise, examine the motives of the messenger.

WATER RETENTION,
SALT'S FAULT

Table salt is one of the most common food seasonings. It is composed of sodium and chloride (NaCl). Both elements are essential to all living organisms. Salt will not release energy when consumed (meaning it cannot make you fatter), but in excess amounts it could increase water retention in the body and cause aesthetic or even health problems. Any food that contains a significant amount of sodium in its natural content can cause water retention, regardless of whether salt has been added during processing, preparation or consumption. The sodium level in a particular food can be found in tables of food contents or on the nutritional label on food packaging.

In practical terms, if you consume sodium-rich food, your body could retain water and make you look fatter and bloated, although your fat level will not be affected. Reducing or eliminating salt from your diet, and choosing foods with lower levels of naturally-occurring sodium, will prevent this from occurring.

This is important to understand when you are considering some fat loss programs, and they suggest you reduce salt intake so you can lose fat faster or more successfully. By doing so you will not benefit your fat loss at all although you might lose a certain amount of water weight and, because of that, reduce your body weight by a few pounds.

When that happens, you might think the world of their diet, but in actuality your fat level is still the same. Reduce your body weight by gradual fat loss due to energy deficit, not water release and dehydration.

Water retention solely due to increased salt intake could increase your body weight by a few percentage points. However, you will not increasingly retain water indefinitely, just because you consume more salt. If you gained 50 pounds over the last year, for example, that is fat, not water retention due to salt intake. Exaggerated water retention can be a body's rebound reaction to dehydration, but that should stabilize fairly quickly. Alternatively, it can be caused by certain health issues.

To illustrate how unimportant salt is for your fat loss, here is a personal example. Generally, I don't have a taste for salt, so I do not add it to my food. However, when I am on a fat loss diet, I put a significant amount of salt on some foods. I do it just because I feel like it (I listen to my body), not because of some medical or fitness reason. Needless to say, in spite of adding salt, I successfully lose fat.

The only time I think about salt and sodium intake is one week before a body building show. Then I reduce sodium to a minimum in order to reveal the maximum potential of my physique. If I did not reduce salt and sodium intake for the show, I would probably have a few pounds of excess retained water, making me look a bit blurry. However, I would still be in good shape, due to fat loss during the previous months.

In this book I state that I often lose 15-20 pounds of body weight due to water release one week before a show. Such intense maneuvering is not achieved just by avoiding salt, but also by other aggressive methods of dehydration and water release. Salt reduction alone would cause a much smaller weight reduction overall.

DEHYDRATION IS NOT
FAT LOSS

For healthy individuals, ingested and eliminated water are in balance. When you distort this balance by forceful water release, the body will try to reestablish it as soon as possible. Body weight that was lost due to dehydration will be gained back rapidly when a sufficient amount of fluid becomes available.

> *Imagine an orange, dried-up on the inside, surrounded by its usual thick peel – not a good way to lose weight.*

In addition, by dehydration you are doing more harm to muscle than to fat because muscle is over 70% water, whereas fat is less than 20% water. A dehydrated person has dramatically lowered physical capabilities, including less strength and endurance.

To give you a better picture of dehydration, imagine an orange, dried-up on the inside, surrounded by its usual thick peel. In a similar way, you can radically dehydrate your body with medications, physical exertion, or extensive use of a sauna, without replacing fluids. If you do that, your muscles and overall body volume will indeed shrink like the inside of the orange, but your skin folds (thickness of your skin and fat) will remain almost unchanged. What that means is that you will now weigh less but have almost the same thick layer of fat covering a smaller, dehydrated lean body mass.

BODY REBOUNDS

The body wants to be in balance and will try to re-establish that balance when it is distorted. The more you distort its balance, the more severe of a rebound you can expect, and the body's health, function and appearance could be jeopardized.

For example, if you distort the body's balance with crash dieting, such as dehydration and starvation, at the first opportunity the body will rebound in proportion to the imposed stress. Meaning, your body weight will be back where it was before such treatment, plus a few more pounds as soon as you start eating and drinking as you normally do. After a while it will likely stabilize back to the initial weight. This is why crash dieting doesn't work. To have lower but stable body weight, you must lose fat gradually, not dehydrate or starve yourself.

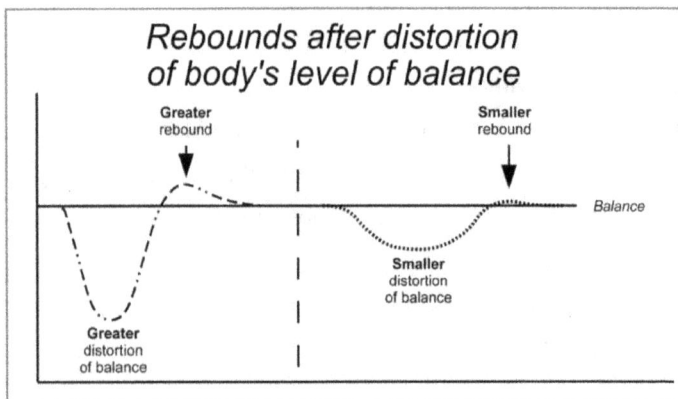

LOSE IT
AND KEEP IT LEAN

It is easier to maintain a desired body condition than to obtain it. However, even for maintenance effort is needed. In the case of fat loss, to lose fat you must be in energy deficit, and to maintain your current level of fat you must be in energy balance. Therefore, to maintain a certain level just continue with whatever you did to lose fat, only a bit less strictly.

The higher the goal you have attained, the harder you will have to work to maintain it. If you dropped your body fat percentage from 25% to only 5%, for example, you will have to be a "slave" to such a remarkable condition.

However, to keep it at 12%, much less effort will be necessary, and you will still be in good condition. I suggest in every fat loss program, either to obtain or maintain your condition, avoid exaggerations. Accept the proper life style that fits you the best, be consistent, and avoid doing things in sudden bursts or on occasion.

SWITCH BACK SLOWLY

When you achieve your desired lower level of body fat, don't go back to your previous lifestyle and let go of the diet and exercise. I've made this mistake more than a few times, and each time I did not like the result. If you go back to a more sedentary lifestyle with an excessive energy intake, the very same lifestyle that made you fat and unhappy before, then your current optimal body condition will soon be ruined and you will be fat and unhappy again. That would be like vacuuming your living room nice and clean, and then emptying your vacuum cleaner bag all over the floor and furniture.

No matter how tempting it may be, do not just say one day, "I am done, now I can eat plenty and stop exercising." Instead, when the fat loss goal is reached, very gradually switch from an obtaining to a maintaining program. It is better to slowly, little by little every week, increase your food intake, and change or decrease your level of physical exercise. That way your body will have enough time to adjust to the new circumstances, and you will have enough time to properly evaluate how these changes influence you.

However, at the end of your fat loss program when you have obtained your desired result, and before you start a maintenance program, give yourself a few days off to reward yourself for achieving success and perhaps to signify the change from one program to another. During those few days, eat as much as you want.

When during your maintenance program you want to take days off, you obviously cannot take them off on the basis of earning them (as described for "Earned days off") because you are not losing any more body weight. You are now maintaining your lean physique with a consistent body weight. Therefore, take a day off when you feel like you need it or schedule it on a certain week day. If you start gaining weight again, that means you are taking too many days off, or your maintenance program between days off is insufficient. For more details on days off, see "Days off and fat loss", page 133-150.

Finally, once you are done losing fat and are no longer motivated by fat loss itself or even by maintaining your new good condition, it is still recommended for your health and general well-being to watch your nutrition and keep exercising.

NEVER GET FAT AGAIN

People talk about fat loss diets, exercises or products that will get you lean, and keep you from ever getting fat again. There is no such thing. No matter how you got in good shape (lost fat, or anything else), you will lose it if you revert back to an inappropriate lifestyle again. However, if it is any consolation, getting in good shape the second time, or any time after, is often easier than getting there in the first place. Still, it is never a cake walk.

CHAPTER FIVE

To pig out or not to pig out? Should you pick a personal trainer for his or her looks, or is there more to it? Do you produce a fat loss dissertation in your fat loss journal, or do you keep it simple, like a to-do list? Is it necessary to use a diabolical egg white and lettuce diet providing seven and a half calories per day, or can you lose fat with a cozier approach? Chapter Five reveals simple and super-efficient ways to make your fat loss easier. It also unveils some of the most practical and efficient shortcuts to use on the way to your leaner self.

HOW STRICT IS THE DIET?

Even though the only determining fat loss factor is eating less energy than you need, I also recommend for health and well-being that you pay attention to the balance of your nutrition, especially consumption of high quality protein. Protein is the body's major building material and, therefore, must be part of any proper nutritional approach, including fat loss. Eating less and consuming properly balanced nutrition are important concepts for fat loss. If you are not familiar with them, I suggest you refer to Chapter Two, page 33-58 and Appendix Two, "Nutrition", page 224-240.

At the beginning of your fat loss diet, you have to evaluate how serious you are about losing fat, and how much time and energy you are willing to invest, or better yet are capable of investing. These are going to be crucial factors for deciding how strict a diet you should use. You also have to decide if you wish to design your own completely original diet, or if you wish to follow diets that are available on the market. You can also mix the two approaches. In any case, following are three options I think you should consider.

Consume smaller meals

If you are not very serious, or do not have much time and energy to invest in your fat loss program, but still want to try it, I suggest you keep eating exactly like you usually do, only one-third less. Simply reduce one-third of each portion of food included in that meal. It is not the same if you reduce two-thirds of the broccoli but leave a whole dessert. Also, when you start reducing one-third of your meals, you cannot increase the number or size of meals. Everything else has to stay the same as before. A fat loss journal will help you track your nutrition and prevent increasing the number or size of your meals.

By eating one-third less you will hopefully create an energy deficit and start losing fat. If you do not notice a fat loss, that means you are still eating too much, so keep further reducing your food intake until desired progress is evident.

This approach to a fat loss diet will not give you the exact knowledge of how many calories you have consumed throughout the day, but if you keep feeling fairly hungry you will lose fat just fine. Keep dieting like this until you drop about 5-10 pounds, depending on your body size. Then, if you wish, switch to a more elaborate approach to fat loss nutrition. Of course, you can keep doing the same thing as long as you keep losing fat, no need to fix something that is not broken.

This method of dieting is less work than strictly controlling your nutrition and keeping a detailed fat loss journal, and therefore many people like it. But for me it does not work. For me eating one-third less of foods I really like requires more self-control than designing a diet of less tasty foods with low calories. Also, not knowing the nutritional facts (because in this method I do not precisely measure my food, and I do not keep a fat loss journal) makes me feel uncomfortable. That is just my personal preference.

You must find what fits you the best. Keep in mind, successful fat loss can be achieved in countless ways, so find or design one that fits your preferences.

Consume smaller meals with lower energy foods

As in the approach I just described, noticeably reduce the size of your meals but also pay closer attention to what you eat. That way you will double the impact on reducing your energy intake. In this approach, you should eliminate energy-rich foods from your menu that you do not really crave, and replace them with lower energy foods.

For instance, instead of eating breakfast with three whole eggs (a total of about 210 calories), eat one whole egg and four egg whites (a total of about 122 calories). That way the meal will taste almost the same, and you will get the same amount of protein, but about 90 calories less. Similarly, in a fast food restaurant, you can order a grilled chicken sandwich. Then, remove the bread (all or just half of the bread), dry off energy-rich seasonings, and eat it with only vegetables. If you do this, you can eat food in a fast food restaurant that is nearly as lean as if you specifically prepared it at home. Even better, many fast food restaurants offer well-balanced but low-energy meals with detailed nutritional information provided at the restaurant or on their websites.

This approach of consuming smaller meals with lower energy foods can carry you far in the fat loss process. Even approximate tracking of calories and protein intake can be done fairly well if you stay away from excessive recipes with unknown nutritional content.

Control your nutrition strictly

This is the most serious approach to fat loss. It includes thoughtful choice of low energy foods, but with necessary nutrients, strict control of the amount of food that is consumed, the leanest methods of food preparation, keeping a detailed fat loss journal, and so on. This approach can be more or less extreme, but if done right always produces great fat loss results. Unlike the previous two approaches, by controlling your nutrition strictly you will have very precise information about the amount of energy and high quality protein consumed throughout the day. Precise information enables you to navigate your fat loss not by guess work, but rather by numbers and facts, as you should.

Caution is needed. If you start your fat loss immediately using this approach, without building up to it, it can be quite a shock. Switching from plentiful and careless eating to a restricted and controlled nutritional plan fits some people, but many give up long before their goal is reached. I almost always approach my fat loss this way, but more than a few times when my motives for losing fat were not strong enough, I gave up after a few days. If you decide to start with this approach, you have to try to overcome the initial shock for at least the first two weeks. It takes a bit of time to adjust to such a drill and maybe even start enjoying it.

TAKE SHORT BREAKS

When intending to eat less, try this. Every time you eat, stop in the middle of your meal for about five to ten minutes. Then, before you continue eating, reevaluate how hungry you really are. Often you will see that even half of your planned meal satiates you and you realistically do not need to eat more. However, if you keep eating without stopping in the middle, you will consume all the food in front of you and might even ask for more before you feel full and satisfied. The body's hunger response is delayed in registering satiation. Therefore, give your body enough time, and do not let the initial impulse of hunger and its momentum control you.

Sometimes when dieting, if you do not have food for a prolonged period of time (such as five hours, for example), you will feel you need a "ton" of food in your next meal to satisfy your hunger. However, often only a few hundred calories will be enough, especially if you eat using the previously described short breaks.

DON'T BE A HERO

In executing your fat loss diet, be realistic and find the approach that fits you the best. Don't try to be a "hero" and do it fast. Fat loss is hard work, and if you overburden yourself, you will probably burn out and give up. Apply gradual changes. If necessary start with the easiest approach, then work your way gradually into more challenging strategies. Especially if you start with a more challenging approach, do not create too great of an energy deficit. Be reasonable. You will be a "hero" if you lose fat, regardless of how fast you did it.

Avoid the typical sickness of our society called *Instant Gratification*. For fat loss, and any other positive change to the body, you have to build results slowly. Progress forward one lost pound at a time, one successful training at a time. Conditioning is a cumulative process. Individually each of those lost pounds or successful trainings do not represent much, but, when added to the positive results of previous lost pounds or trainings, amazing changes are to be expected.

THE DRUG-ADDICT, ALCOHOLIC AND SMOKER

Keep the following extreme example in mind when you start incorporating changes into your lifestyle. If you were a drug-addict, alcoholic and smoker, you would not try to drop all three addictions at once. If you did, there is a big chance your efforts would collapse under the shock of such radical change. You would need to quit gradually. First you could stop using drugs. Then, when you adjusted to that, you could stop drinking. Finally, after you adjusted to the absence of alcohol, you could then stop smoking.

The same goes for changes you apply regarding losing fat. If you are physically passive and tend to overeat, do not try to change both at once. For most people it is better if they incorporate changes gradually. If you are the same way, first start exercising. Then, after your body gets used to it and gets over the initial muscle soreness, incorporate a fat loss diet, or vice versa. Give yourself enough time to be ready for a new change, and set yourself up to win.

ENERGY RATIOS

Energy ratios of nutrients are different depending on the type of diet and source of information you wish to consider. Keep in mind these ratios refer to percentages of energy, not percentages of grams. Fat releases more than twice the amount of energy than proteins and carbohydrates compared gram to gram.

	Carb %	Prot %	Fat %
Common medical recommendation	55	15	30
Moderate diet	50	25	25
Low fat diet	60	25	15
Low carb diet	10	45	45
My usual fat loss diet	45 to 65	25 to 45	10

You can see that energy ratios are all over the board as you go from one type of diet to another. Until you discover what fits you the best, use percentages for the "Common medical recommendation" or the "Moderate diet". Even better, ask for professional help regarding ratios most suitable for you. Energy ratios of nutrients are good guidelines to provide your body with a variety of foods for optimal healthy and balanced nutrition, as well as improved taste. However, for fat loss alone, ratios of nutrients are irrelevant. Some people think they will lose fat faster if they count grams of carbs or fats, pay attention to the structure of carbs or fats, cycle carbs or fats, or follow other types of trendy, prescribed fads. These methods are purely a waste of time. What is going to make you lose fat is energy deficit, regardless of how you mix nutrients.

RECENT DISCOVERY
OF OLD NEWS

I recently came across another fat loss "breakthrough". In one book published in 2009 the authors stated, "Recent studies have shown that diets with extra protein are more satisfying and result in greater weight loss". However, more than a half century ago, bodybuilders all over the world were already using diets higher in protein to lower their body fat. Even then it was old news, and now recent studies have finally "discovered the truth"! I am anxiously awaiting another "recent study" to finally discover the truth about which side of the world we can expect the sun to come up in the morning!

> *We are not fat due to misunderstanding nutritional details, or because we did not read the latest scientific research. We are fat because we eat too much. Period.*

We are not fat due to misunderstanding nutritional details, or because we did not read the latest scientific research reinventing the wheel. We are fat because we eat too much, period. There is no energy ratio of nutrients that will make you not want to eat too much when you diet. Even a high protein diet will not contribute to fat loss if you eat too much. The urge to eat more than you really require is created by your mind. Therefore, eat whichever ratio of nutrients fits you the best, but control your mind, and you will lose fat.

USE ANY COLOR YOU LIKE

When I am not on a fat loss program, both now and when I competed in the past, I pay very little attention to what I eat. I eat whatever I like in the approximate amount that I need. Apart from trying to have high quality protein in most of my meals, I do not know how many calories or grams of protein I consume, nor do I know my energy ratios. However, if I start getting too fat, I eat less or restart my fat loss diet, and remedy it.

When I competed, people used to ask me why I was so relaxed during off season, eating "forbidden" things, when most of my colleagues watched their nutritional intake religiously all the time. There is a very simple reason: I was involved in competitive bodybuilding for almost twenty years, and I wanted to make it easier on myself. I did not want to live 12 months of the year like I was in prison measuring every bite I ate. What kind of life would that be? All that hardship, just to avoid gaining a few extra pounds of fat.

By eating casually during my off season, I usually gained no more than 10-15 pounds of excess weight. It was easier for me to be on my diet a few weeks longer, and lose those extra pounds of fat during that time, than to stress out about my nutrition the remaining eight months of the year (I was usually dieting for competition four months of the year).

I am not saying this is the way you should do it. Many fat loss guides advise you to be uptight in one way or another, so I am simply telling you that you can actually relax and make fat loss more humane. This book is teaching you the right way to hold the brush while you paint the portrait of your own fat loss. What colors to use is entirely up to you.

PAY MORE ATTENTION

As opposed to times I am not on a fat loss program, when it comes to composing and executing my fat loss diet, I pay close attention to and control my calorie and protein intake very strictly. Again, though, I do not pay attention to the energy ratios of nutrients at all. I pick foods that will serve my fat loss needs the best, and compose meals and menus from them considering overall energy and protein intake. I also try to have at least some variety, for taste as well as more balanced nutrition. The reason I include the energy ratios of nutrients here is because during my career I had to analyze my diets for public presentations, lectures and books. Since some people subscribe to the use of energy ratios for fat loss, I needed to address it. Otherwise, for practical fat loss purposes, energy ratios do not mean much.

Most people do not know about energy ratios including their protein or caloric intake. Ask a number of both lean and fat people around you; I doubt that one out of ten will know a single one of those values. The fact that they do not know will not make them fat. I promote paying attention to your protein intake and proper nutritional balance, but you can lose fat by energy deficit alone, even if you don't eat protein or any other nutrient for that matter. Even

> *Pay attention to protein intake, but for fat loss alone energy deficit is all you need.*

though you can eat the most unhealthy of foods and still lose fat, don't. You do not want to just lose fat, you want to lose fat and stay strong and healthy too. That is why you should give your body a variety of foods while keeping your energy intake at a suitable level for fat loss.

PROTEIN CALORIES STAY THE SAME, THE REST CHANGES

In summary: for your fat loss diet if you wish to control your nutrition strictly and pay attention to your energy intake and quantity of high quality protein consumption, you could benefit from the following guidelines. These guidelines are simplified, so if you decide to apply them, use reason and flexibility.

Protein energy intake

Protein needs may be different from one person to another depending on various factors. For more details see "Proteins, energy-rich nutrients", page 225-230. However, once your specific needs for high quality protein are determined, you can consider them constant, and they have to be met regularly. Such needs will be constant until some radical and fairly permanent change happens in your circumstances. For instance, the amount of your daily physical activity could change, or you could experience a significant change in body weight. At that time identify your new protein needs and keep them constant until circumstances change again.

You do not need to change your protein intake just because one day you increase your physical activity due to shoveling a driveway after a snow storm or because you gain five pounds when you pigged out last night. Adjusting protein consumption due to such sporadic and short-lasting change is not necessary or practical.

Also, you do not need to eat exactly the same amount of protein every day. Just keep yourself fairly close to the recommended intake, even if you miss it by a few grams. If you wish, you can eat more protein than your daily requirement. That will not hurt your health or fat loss, as long as you are moderate and stay within your energy intake limits.

Carbohydrate energy intake

Carbohydrate intake can be larger or smaller each day, depending on the level of physical activity of the particular day. For example, if you had to shovel snow off your driveway, you can consume more carbohydrates that day, unlike with proteins which you do not need to adjust (but you can if you want to). However, to supply your body with more energy you can eat any energy-rich nutrient, not only carbohydrates.

Fat energy intake

Fat is to be kept low during a fat loss diet, not because its energy is especially dangerous for fat loss, but because if you consume one gram of fat, you have already ingested an amount equivalent to about 2.25 grams of proteins or carbohydrates. By eating more grams of fat, you will

> *Low carb diets are media-created diversions to proper thinking about fat loss.*
> ***
> *Carbs and fats don't make you fat. Too many calories do, regardless of where they come from!*

have fewer grams of protein and carbohydrates available before you reach your desired daily energy intake. That means less food and probably fewer, smaller meals. However, if you crave a particular food with a high level of fat, eat it regardless of its ratio of nutrients, but stay within your energy limits. *Excess energy from fat is no more dangerous for your fat loss than the same excess amount coming from any other nutrient.*

Since protein needs are essentially constant every day, we can conclude that every day we should consume the same amount of energy coming from protein. The rest of the energy can come from any kind of nutrient (carbohydrates, fats or even more protein than your required amount if you wish), irrespective of their ratios.

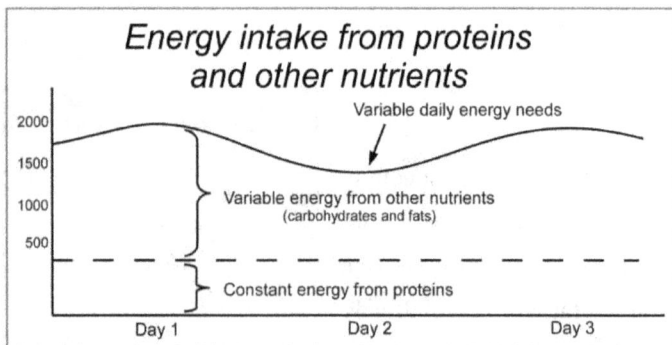

Energy intake from proteins and other nutrients

Variable daily energy needs

Variable energy from other nutrients (carbohydrates and fats)

Constant energy from proteins

Day 1   Day 2   Day 3

HOW MANY CALORIES?

If you decide to lose fat by controlling your nutrition strictly, you will diet by numbers. Numbers will give you the facts, a solid sense of direction while you navigate through your fat loss. If you do not navigate by numbers, there is a good chance that you will either consume too many calories or too few (the same goes for grams of protein). If you consume too many calories, you will not lose fat and may even get fatter. If you consume too few calories, you will burn out and compromise the success of your fat loss.

I am often asked, "How many calories should I eat to lose fat?" The only true answer is, "You should consume fewer calories than you need to maintain your current body weight." When dieting for fat loss by numbers, you typically need to establish the number of calories you need each day to maintain your current body weight. That is your energy maintenance level. From that number of calories you have to set your desired energy deficit. The most suitable energy deficit is about 20% less energy than your maintenance level. Such deficit should produce fairly fast fat loss results without excessive stress.

If you want faster or slower fat loss, create a greater or smaller energy deficit, respectively, and see how it works for you. I usually create a greater energy deficit during my diets, just to speed it up and get it over with sooner.

DETERMINING CALORIE NEEDS

These are a few tools and methods you can use to determine your energy needs, and, from there, identify the energy deficit needed for fat loss.

Instruments

You can use instruments to calculate your daily energy needs. Some instruments will measure your basal metabolic rate (BMR), but they cannot predict how much energy you will need for all activities during the day. Other instruments are affixed to the body to cumulatively register daily spent energy. Every 24 hours you can check results. To use this type of instrument most effectively, you should wear it for a few or more days, to gain a more accurate idea about your average energy needs, because you do not spend the same amount of energy every day. Some users suggest wearing these instruments for a week because they notice a difference in energy expenditure up to 30-40% between workdays and weekends. Once you know how much energy you usually spend each day, keep your nutrition at an energy deficit that suits you the best.

Take the results of these instruments as guidelines only. As with all methods, and regularly throughout your fat loss, evaluate how the numbers or applied programs are working for your fat loss, and then correct them if needed.

Literature

You can consult specialized literature, the Internet or other sources for an approximate idea of how many calories a person of your specifications would need to maintain or lose body weight. There are also various formulas out there to help you calculate your energy needs.

Manual calculation

You can manually calculate your energy needs. To do so, you have to carefully calculate and log calories of everything you eat and drink during a period of at least 10 days. Next you add all these calories together and divide that number by the number of days that you have been counting calories (10, in our example). The result is your average energy intake per day. During these 10 days, try not to change your usual daily routine, especially with regard to physical activity.

Weigh yourself at the beginning and at the end of the 10 days. If you gained one pound, that means in the last 10 days you had a total excess energy of about 3500 calories, 350 calories per day too much. If you lost one pound over the 10-day period, you had 3500 calories too little, an energy deficit of 350 calories per day. If you stayed the same weight during the 10 days, you have been consuming the exact amount of energy that you needed.

Do not apply this method for periods shorter than 10 days, because body weight oscillations can be due to other reasons, and that can confuse you. To get results that are as accurate as possible regarding your initial and final body weight, weigh yourself three days prior and three days after your 10-day test period and calculate the average value. That should minimize the influence of normal body weight oscillations and further reduce confusion.

I have used this manual method a few times during my career, and I do not think the results justify the effort. However, some people appreciate a high level of detail and rigor; they might prefer this method. Also, it can be good practice in keeping an accurate fat loss journal, and in thinking about fat loss through energy deficit in relation to the number of consumed and spent calories.

Guess work

My favorite method of determining optimal energy deficit for fat loss is just to guess the number of calories required and try it out. In the majority of cases I start women on a diet of between 1000 to 1500 calories per day and men between 1500 to 2500 calories each day. Especially women often tell me I started them a bit too high, and I do that on purpose. I think it is better to slowly reduce energy intake than to start too aggressively and scare someone away from fat loss.

It is considered that the average daily energy needs (to maintain current body weight) of women are about 1700 calories, and of men are about 2500 calories.

EVALUATING CALORIE INTAKE

Whichever method you use to calculate or guess your daily energy requirements to lose fat, you have to test the results. You should not just take your initial number for granted, because the initial expectation can be inaccurate.

To explain how to evaluate if a certain caloric intake is appropriate for fat loss, we will consider an example of an overweight male that has an estimated requirement of 2500 calories per day to maintain his current body weight. In order to lose fat, he should reduce his energy intake by about 20% from the estimated 2500 calories. Therefore, he should be consuming about 2000 calories per day. That will create an energy deficit of 500 calories per day. Following are a few scenarios explaining what to do both in the case where 2000 calories per day is the appropriate energy intake, or inappropriate energy intake for him to lose fat.

We will disregard the initial quantum weight drop that happens at the beginning of a fat loss diet and consider fat loss and weight loss that happens after the first few days.

2000 calories - good energy intake

If 2000 calories is a good energy intake, he will lose fat (weight) gradually, but still fast enough. He will be slightly hungry and tired, however in very good physical and mental shape. He will be able to maintain fat loss long enough to accomplish his goal. As long as he keeps losing fat in this way, he doesn't need to change anything. When his body adapts to that energy level intake and fat loss starts to slow down or even stop, he will have to start consuming less or spending more energy.

This is an example of the right way to lose fat. In this scenario, our subject will lose an average of about one pound of fat each week, because one pound of fat contains about 3500 calories. He was in an energy deficit of 500 calories each day for seven days. That equals 3500 calories of total deficit for the week. Do not get stuck on one pound per week. As long as you feel good while losing fat, you can lose less or more.

2000 calories - too low of an energy intake

If 2000 calories is too low of an energy intake, our guy will lose fat (weight) fast, but he will soon start experiencing negative symptoms such as feeling overly hungry, chronically weak and tired, sleepless, unable to focus and keep up with daily work, an aggravated and aggressive attitude, and so on. Such symptoms are problematic, in spite of fast and obvious fat loss.

To overcome this problem, I suggest increasing energy intake by 500 calories per day. That is, he should consume 2500 calories per day. That also means the initial assumption was wrong, and his maintenance energy level is higher than 2500 calories. Such mistakes happen often and can be easily corrected. At this point, while consuming 2500 calories per day, if he keeps losing fat and feeling as described above in the first scenario, then that is a good energy intake for him. If he still does not feel good enough after the first increase in 500 calories, he should keep increasing his energy intake little by little until he feels good enough yet keeps losing fat. If he stops losing fat, he is eating too much.

Any person on a fat loss diet will feel a bit hungry and tired, maybe even aggravated because of the necessary energy deficit. Energy intake cannot be increased just to make a person feel great. Fat loss is the criteria, and some reasonable discomfort comes with the territory.

> *During fat loss, get used to being a bit hungry. Energy intake cannot be increased just to make a person feel great. Losing fat is what matters.*

Usually, when energy intake is increased or decreased, I suggest a 10-day trial period because necessary adaptations are not instantly obvious. However, sometimes changes can be made after much shorter periods if there is an obvious need for doing so. For example, if you started your fat loss with far too low of an energy intake, it would be too stressful to continue for another 10 days to prove something that was obviously wrong from the beginning.

2000 calories - too high of an energy intake

If 2000 calories is too high of an energy intake, during the first 10 days our guy will not lose fat (weight). In this case, I suggest decreasing energy intake by 500 calories. He should keep this lower energy intake of 1500 calories each day for about 10 days and watch for new developments. If he starts losing fat and feels as described above for "good energy intake" for fat loss, he should continue like this until fat loss stops or slows down. If he still does not lose a noticeable amount of fat after 10 days on 1500 calories per day, then energy intake should again be decreased by approximately 500 calories per day (now he would be consuming 1000 calories per day). At this point, if he is not losing fat, he is most likely lying about his daily calorie intake, and he should track it accurately and also keep reducing it until he starts losing fat.

UNDER-REPORTING CALORIES

In many cases people under-report their calorie intake because they do not log everything in their fat loss journal. They forgot to include a few snacks in the calculation. If and when you decide to control your nutrition strictly and count your calories, you have to be very accurate in logging everything you consume; otherwise there is no point in doing it. If you are not going to be accurate, don't waste your time weighing, calculating and logging your food.

SHIFTING CALORIES UP AND DOWN

When you determine your energy level for fat loss, you do not need to stick with the exact number every day. Adjust it up and down a bit, depending on your mental state and physical condition each day. For example, your basic plan is to consume 2000 calories per day to lose fat. When you start, you can consume energy like this: 2000, 2100, 2050, 1800, 1900, 2075, and so on. Along the same line of thinking, energy deficit does not always have to be 20%. Rather, you can shift it to 15%, 30%, 25% and so on.

The fat loss rule is to stay mostly in energy deficit, occasionally in energy balance, and very rarely in energy surplus.

Also, do not force yourself to eat the planned number of calories if you do not need them, eat less. The next day you could need to eat a bit more. Play around with your numbers to satisfy your body and mind, but make sure you are still losing fat. The fat loss rule is to stay mostly within an energy deficit, occasionally in energy balance, and very rarely in energy surplus.

Do not get too aggressive on your diet unless you must for an important deadline. No need to rush anything. Lose fat gradually, step by step. Ten small and safe steps will get you further than one huge jump ending with a broken leg.

FAT LOSS JOURNAL – NAVIGATE BY COMPASS, NOT BY BREEZE

The fat loss journal is the most important tool in dieting by numbers. If you don't diet by numbers, you diet by feelings. This is like trying to sail to a specific location by following

> *A fat loss journal will change your outlook on fatness and fat loss forever.*
> *It's hard to fool yourself when you see the truth.*

the breeze, rather than navigating by a compass. It is possible to lose fat without keeping a fat loss journal, but the power of keeping a fat loss journal is one of the key messages you should get from this book, and it greatly increases your chances of success. Most likely it will open your eyes, and you will see facts about dieting entirely differently than you did before.

Think about it similarly to how you track finances. You should not simply guess at your income and expenses. You need to keep precise records and update them on a regular basis in order to know your financial condition. A fat loss journal does the same thing for your diet.

A fat loss journal is an especially important tool for people who strictly control their food intake during fat loss. Even people that are not on such a strict program can benefit from a fat loss journal. These are some reasons that make a fat loss journal such an important tool:

- It will enable you daily to lose fat by numbers and recorded facts, not by feelings and guesses, which are often very deceiving. At the end of every day you will know exactly how many calories and grams of high quality protein you consumed. This information is the backbone of the most effective diets.

- It will provide records that can be used retroactively to track your progress, and to analyze the efficiency of your fat loss program throughout its different stages.

- Just the fact that you are paying such close attention to your food consumption and logging it in your journal, will stop you from deviating from your program, and doing a "bad thing" that could harm your fat loss.

- It will keep you motivated by showing all the work you have invested in fat loss, especially if progress is obvious. Even without progress, it will make you feel like you do not want to give up after all that work already invested. You will want to continue and make changes to start achieving progress.

INFORMATION TO RECORD

There is no need for fancy pre-designed journals. A simple notebook will do just fine. Whatever you use, make sure it is durable, because you will be opening it maybe 10 times per day for the next few months or longer. Use something with a substantial amount of space on each page and plenty of pages, because recordings will accumulate into a lot of information. Many people use computers or cellular phones as fat loss journals. I think old fashioned recording on a piece of paper will give you better visualization of your diet.

The idea of a fat loss journal is to record data for current and future use. You do not need to do sophisticated statistical calculations in order to feel like you are using your journal and recorded data. It is often enough just to glance through at the end of the day to check your numbers, or maybe reflect on something that happened yesterday.

Record everything that can help you. Whatever you decide to log in, make sure it is recorded completely and accurately. Also, keep your records clear and easy to read, don't just write something that no one, including you, will be able to decipher later.

Following is what I think you should record in a fat loss journal.

Date and total days of losing fat

For example, if I started my fat loss diet on Sunday 01/01/2006, I would log that date, and next to it the number one, representing my first day of losing fat. Months later, I would put Friday 04/21/2006 which represents a current date, and next to it number 111 which would be my total number of days losing fat as of that day. If I have a deadline ahead of me, I can add the number of the days remaining until my deadline to the number of days that I already have been dieting. If I have 120 days to lose fat, the first day of my diet I would write 1/119, and as time goes by, the numbers would change to 119/1, representing that I already dieted for 119 days and have one more day to finish my diet.

Body weight and other body measurements

I usually record my body weight in the morning, or sometimes in the gym before my workout. Every two weeks, or once a month, I also record circumference measurements and body fat percentages.

Nutrition

This is the most important part of the fat loss journal because nothing comes even close to the influence of nutrition on fatness and fat loss. When you record your nutrition, I suggest you log the following information.

- *Time of each meal.* Every time you put something in your mouth that has calories, that is, food or drink, write down the exact time. That will give you an idea of how your meals are spread out, and the time gaps between consumption of proteins and energy during the day.

- *Type and amount of food consumed in each meal.* This information will enable you to calculate two very important things: the amount of high quality protein and the amount of calories consumed in each meal.

- *The exact number of grams of high quality protein and amount of calories for each meal, and the day in total.* This information allows you to see your actual consumption compared to your planned protein and energy intake.

  In your fat loss journal, you only record grams of high quality protein. Grams of low quality protein are not recorded. Foods that contain low quality protein will be considered and recorded in your journal exclusively for the energy they provide. On the other hand, foods that contain high quality protein will be considered and recorded for both energy and grams of protein they provide. See "Proteins, energy-rich nutrients", page 225-230.

- *Ratio between total number of meals and meals with high quality protein.* When dieting for fat loss one of the things you could be missing is high quality protein. To eliminate that risk, I recommend you incorporate high quality protein into almost all of your meals. That is why recording ratios of total meals and meals with high quality protein can come handy. For instance, if you had a total of five meals with only one meal containing high quality protein, you have to increase the number of protein-rich meals. But if you had a total of five meals, and four meals had high quality protein, changes are probably not needed.

Physical exercise

When it comes to training, I usually record only the basics. However, more detailed notes could be useful, especially in the beginning. You could log how many trainings you had, how long they lasted, if you used resistance training or cardio, which resistance exercises you used, how long and what type of cardio exercise you used, and so on.

Other relevant information

In your fat loss journal you can also record days off, health conditions, pictures of progress, overall mood, planned changes, and anything else relevant to your fat loss process.

Time and time again, I hear the same feedback from my clients. After they keep a fat loss journal for the first time, they come to me shocked with their revelations about their own daily nutritional intake. Even if you initially decide to lose fat without a journal, I suggest you try it at least for a week, precisely logging and calculating everything. You too will never see fat loss the same way again.

> *Without a fat loss journal, you only guess and hope for the best.*

The following is an example of my fat loss journal.

240 lbs

SUNDAY 01/01/2006 (1/119)

		PROTEIN	CALORIES
7:15am)	3 EGGS	18	210
	3 EGG WHITES	9	39
	170g TOMATO	/	31
	1 YOGURT	6	110
	250g APPLE	/	130
		33	520
10:30am)	1 YOGURT	6	110
	125g (½) APPLE	/	65
		6	175
1:30 pm)	200g COTTAGE CHEESE	24	142
	80g RICE	/	288
	125g (½) APPLE	/	65
		24	495
4:30 pm)	1½ SCOOPS OF PROTEIN POWDER	30	180
8:00 pm)	8 EGG WHITES	24	104
	50g RICE	/	180
	1 YOGURT	6	110
	125g (½) APPLE	/	65
		30	459

(5/5) TOTAL FOR DAY: 123g 1829cal

WORKOUT   1. RESISTANCE TRAINING
5:30-7pm   (ARMS, SHOULDERS, ABDOMINALS)
                   2. CARDIO EXERCISE - WALKING

DAYS OFF AND FAT LOSS

I am a big fan and promoter of days off during a fat loss program. The idea is that you stick with your fat loss program strictly, but periodically take a day off. On your day off, you generally consume more and a greater variety of foods, and typically don't exercise. That way you break your total fat loss into smaller portions which are individually easier to handle, rather than going all the way to the end without any breaks.

Personally, I don't like dieting at all, so I put up with my program very strictly for a shorter period of time, then take a day off and relax. Alternating it like this makes it much easier and more efficient for me. After a day off, I feel physically stronger and more motivated for further fat loss. Days off are not a must but can be a very useful tool. If days off are not taken, there is a chance you will become too saturated with the fat loss process, and its effectiveness will fade, or that you may even give up.

CHEATING DAYS

Some people refer to days off as "cheating days". Essentially, who cares what you call them, as long as you apply them correctly. However, if you could cheat and actually lose fat, I would be the first one doing it all these years. I, too, like things to be easy and comfortable. If days off are the result of careful planning and successful execution, they work. If they are the result of guilty sneaking and cheating, they don't.

EARNED DAYS OFF

An earned day off is an excellent example of careful planning and successful execution. It can be explained like this. You started your fat loss with a body weight of 185 pounds. Ten days later you lost seven pounds and now your body weight is 178 pounds. Let us say that is on Sunday morning. That Sunday you want to reward yourself for your initial success and take a day off. Eat plenty and do not exercise. Monday morning your body weight may have risen to 181 pounds. Then you start again with your usual fat loss diet and exercise program. How much higher your body weight is after a day off depends on many factors and is likely to be different after each day off. In this example I used an increment of three pounds, but it can be much more or even less.

The next day off is not to be taken as long as your body weight does not reach a level lower than your previous best result. This is the key to an earned day off. You are not rewarded until your weight is lower than before. In this case you would not take a new day off until your body weight reached 176 pounds or lower. After that day off (when you reach 176 pounds), you do not take your next day off until your body weight is 174 pounds, and so on. Days should be taken off in this manner, on an earned basis. You set smaller goals and when you reach them you reward yourself. But you are not to forcefully lower your body weight just to have a day off (for example, by dehydration). Your targeted body weight must happen by following your regular fat loss program.

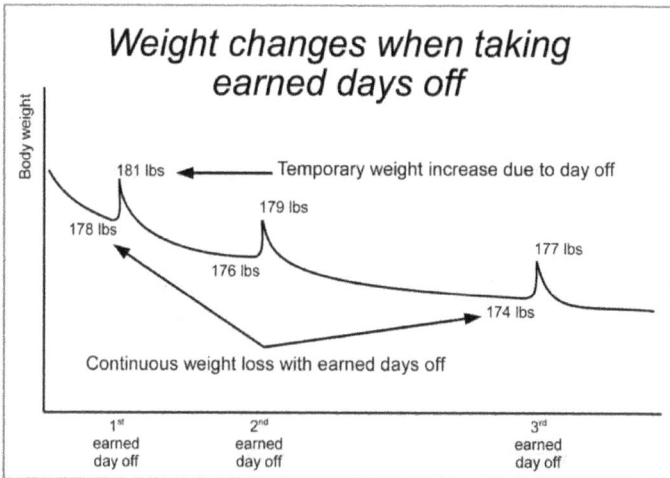

Weight changes when taking earned days off

Body weight

181 lbs ◄———————— Temporary weight increase due to day off

179 lbs

178 lbs

176 lbs

177 lbs

174 lbs

Continuous weight loss with earned days off

1st earned day off | 2nd earned day off | 3rd earned day off

How much of a body weight reduction to set as a goal before taking a next earned day off is an individual choice. I suggest being moderate. A very low goal could be accomplished too soon, and a very high goal could take too long. In most cases it is best to stay in the range of 1-3 pounds of improvement between days off. Also, your earned days off will not occur with regularity. Some will be earned after five days and some could take longer. Furthermore, if you feel you do not need a day off when you reach your goal, don't take it. Lose a few more pounds and then take a day off when you really need it and have earned it even more. On the other hand, if you have an emergency (feel sick, weak, tired, and so on), take a day off even if your targeted body weight has not been reached. However, do not abuse this suggestion and start finding supposed frequent "emergencies".

SCHEDULED DAYS OFF

Different than earning a day off, sometimes people just schedule a day off without earning it. In my opinion that is not the best idea. Here is why.

We will assume you scheduled days off every Sunday, regardless of your body weight improvement. As in the previous example for earned days off, let us say Sunday morning your body weight is 178 pounds, and you take a day off. Monday morning your body weight is back up to 181 pounds. You go back on your diet and you exercise, but do not drop your weight any lower than 179 pounds by next Sunday, which is your next scheduled day off. You take your day off anyway, but at one pound more than last Sunday, and Monday morning you are 182 pounds (one pound more than last Monday). If you keep repeating this sequence, you will end up gaining instead of losing weight. Such an occurrence cannot happen when you take days off on the basis of an accomplished result rather than just a preset schedule.

This example of gaining weight with scheduled days off is a simplified scenario to make the point that scheduled days off are not necessarily efficient. In reality, with scheduled days off, you are more likely not to lose weight than to actually gain weight. When people know that they have a guaranteed scheduled day off, like every Sunday, many will scarcely diet or train during the week. I call this the "alibi diet". However, when a day off is to be earned, most will work even harder than usual to hit the mark and perhaps have a day off earlier than expected. We all are more or less wired that way. Knowing this, we have to set rules that will force us to reach our goal, in this case by using earned rather than scheduled days off.

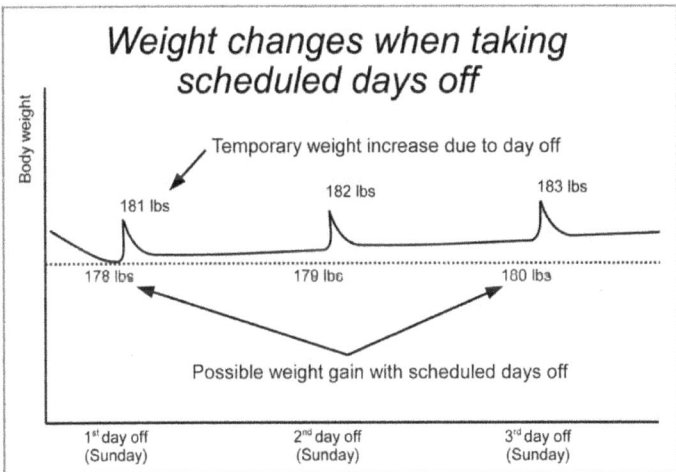

Weight changes when taking scheduled days off

Body weight

Temporary weight increase due to day off

181 lbs

182 lbs

183 lbs

178 lbs

179 lbs

180 lbs

Possible weight gain with scheduled days off

1st day off (Sunday)

2nd day off (Sunday)

3rd day off (Sunday)

SEMI DAYS OFF

A "usual day off", which is an earned, scheduled, or even accidental day off, typically includes excessive consumption of any kind of food, even "fattening" food. Unlike a usual day off without limitations in the amount and type of food, a semi day off includes a slight increase in consumption of the same type of food that is normally consumed during the fat loss program. Semi days off are a great concept, but they mostly serve to rejuvenate the body rather than the mind. Your body will recover from a "few" hundred calories more, however, your mind cares much more about pigging out on "forbidden fruits". For example, if you typically consume 2000 calories during one standard fat loss day, on a semi day off you can consume 3000 calories by eating the same foods.

If you think semi days off are appropriate for you, use them by all means. I suggest taking them off on an earned (or emergency) basis. Also, you do not have to sign a "10 year contract" stating you will exclusively use either semi or usual days off. Use them both as seems appropriate. Unlike taking usual days off, after semi days off your body weight should barely increase.

Some people during fat loss like to increase their energy intake every three to five days (but for one day only), eating exactly the same food as during their normal fat loss program. By increasing calorie intake in this manner, they hope to prevent the body's adjustment to a lower energy intake. Meaning, just about when the body "decides" to lower its energy needs, they confuse it by raising energy intake for only one day. Then, they go back on the lower energy intake. This is very similar to taking semi days off. I have written about this technique and tried it myself. However, these days I do not utilize this approach. First, I cannot really determine if it is effective or not; second, it doesn't provide me with the benefits of a usual, earned day off.

ACCIDENTAL DAYS OFF

I previously explained days off that are planned as part of your fat loss. However, nearly all of us in a fat loss program slip and lose control of our diet, and end up taking an unplanned, "accidental" day off. We must at least try to keep such accidental days off to a minimum. When you do, in fact, slip out of control and have such a day off, do the same as you would do with any other usual day off. Eat, relax and don't worry. When you get back on your diet, everything will return to normal quickly.

NO DAYS OFF

Some people would rather not take days off, usually because of the resultant weight gain. They feel it throws them off rhythm or that it slows down their progress. Taking an earned day off will not make you gain fat, but it will postpone your progress for a day or so because during the day off you were not in energy deficit. You do not need to take days off to have successful fat loss. They are nothing but another available tool to reach your fat loss goal. If you do not need them, do not use them.

THREE CONSECUTIVE DAYS OFF

After a longer period of successful fat loss (e.g. 20 days or longer), up to three consecutive days off can be taken without noticeable accumulation of additional fat. After three days off you should immediately go back on your fat loss program or you will start noticing an increase in fat deposits.

For example, at the beginning of 2002 I started my fat loss diet with a body weight of a bit over 250 pounds. After about two months when my body weight was exactly 200 pounds, I took three consecutive days off (Friday, Saturday and Sunday). During those days I consumed large amounts of food and did not work out at all. This is what happened.

- March 8th 2002 (Friday 7 am), before I started eating I was 200 pounds.

- March 10th 2002 (Sunday 9 pm) after eating and not training for almost three days I was 220 pounds.

- March 11th 2002 (Monday morning) I started with my fat loss routine again.

- March 14th 2002 (Thursday 7 am) I was back to 200 pounds (see page 58).

In other words, in less than a week I went from 200 pounds up to 220 pounds and came back down to 200 pounds. During that time my fat level did not change noticeably. It probably did change a few "grams" but that was not noticeable. My skin folds were the same during all that time, regardless of drastic weight changes.

One of the good points of this example is, even if your body weight increases rapidly after your day or days off, do not worry about it too much. When you get back to your usual fat loss routine, soon everything will be back to normal. Any weight gain or loss that happens suddenly, for example in a day, or two or three, is not related to fat gain or loss.

However, I suggest you do not take more than one well-earned day off at a time, at least until you learn how your body responds. Once in a while, for example, over a long weekend trip out of town, you might take a three-day break without fat gain consequences. Even more ideally, if you don't have cravings during that weekend, don't pig out. Eat anything you want, but reduce portions and it will be as if you have been following your regular fat loss program all along. As I stated before, fat loss or fatness is not related to food choices, but rather the number of calorics you consume.

LOSING RHYTHM

Inexperienced individuals will feel guilty or even panic because of the increased body weight that follows a day off. This is not necessary because as I said before, this body weight increase comes from water and food retention, not actual fat gain. Skipping a workout will also contribute to weight gain, not due to unburned calories, which is a common misconception, but rather due to lack of sweating out the usual amount of fluid which is now retained in the body.

When your body weight increases after a day off, simply go back on your usual fat loss program, and your weight will shortly be back to what it was before. The body weight will be back to normal approximately three days after you stop overeating. It will take about three days regardless if you have taken one or three days off.

> *Don't panic or guilt yourself – body weight increases from retention of food and water, not from fat gain.*

When you take a day off, you will lose "the rhythm" and thwart your fat loss, but only for a short period of time. The body does not need to burn stored fat as long as enough energy is available from food consumption. Once you recreate energy deficit, your body will start burning stored fat again. That will happen even before your body weight comes back down to what it was before you took a day off.

HOW MUCH PIGGING OUT?

I am often asked, "But how much can I really eat on a day off and not get fat the next day?" You really can eat as much as you want or can fit into your stomach. I like to tell my clients, "You really can eat like a swine." It is completely irrelevant what and how much you consume during your day off. If you earned your day off, even if you load yourself with ice cream, cheesecake, chocolate and pizza all day long, you will not store any obvious fat. You will only temporarily gain body weight. I know it is hard to believe, but try it and you will see. Naturally, if you keep taking days off without properly earning them, you will start getting fatter and fatter.

When I was younger on my days off during or even right after those ferocious competitive-driven diets, I used to eat so much that I couldn't breathe properly or bend forward. Not even opening the top button on my pants would help. Right after one show in London, I was eating with a group of friends and one of them remarked, "I cannot believe it, you must have eaten at least 20,000 calories this evening, and you still keep eating like you are hungry". He was probably very close to being accurate about my calorie intake. The very next morning, we had a photo shoot, and I appeared even leaner than on the day of the show (before taking a day off). I did not gain any recognizable fat, even by such gluttony.

I do not recommend that level of excess, but if your mind needs a break, let it have a break and know that even after obnoxious pigging out, even if it lasts for three days, you still don't have to worry about gaining obvious fat. On an earned day off relax and eat freely.

GUILTY FEELING

During a day off, the best thing you can do is to forget about fat loss and eat and drink as much as you want of whatever you want. Don't guilt or limit yourself, because if you do, you will not refresh your mind properly, and that defeats the purpose of a usual day off.

After a day off, a guilty feeling can be useful for more efficient fat loss. If you feel guilty and want to compensate for "damage done" (even though there is no real damage), fat loss nutrition and exercise can be applied more strictly than before. This strict application is beneficial if done within reason, but is not beneficial if it is overdone. Applying too strict of a fat loss program could easily cause overwhelming stress, resulting in burning out and taking another, premature day off.

I used to make that mistake. Specifically, after my day off I was not very hungry, so I hardly ate anything, resulting in overwhelming hunger the following day. It was much better if I started eating my usual fat loss amount after my day off, even if I was not very hungry. That helped me avoid the overwhelming hunger the following day, and I had fewer problems regaining my fat loss rhythm after a day off.

Figuratively speaking, after a day off, it would be better to be 20% stricter than usual and endure it for two weeks, than 50% stricter, and achieve burn out in two days. Do not push your body too far from the state of balance. Sometimes, having too much desire can be harmful to your fat loss, so you have to tame it down a bit.

EXAMPLES OF DAYS OFF

In the following examples, you can see different applications of days off. Some represent good usage, others do not. You will also see the inherent flexibility of the generally recommended principles associated with days off.

Earned evening off

A twenty-eight year old girl started her fat loss program to reach a body weight of 125 pounds. After initial hesitation, she decided to take earned days off every time she decreased her body weight by two pounds. Even though she knew why it happened, her increased body weight after a day off bothered her a lot. To reduce the problem, I suggested she start eating more after 7 pm until she went to bed (but no later than midnight), instead of taking a whole day off. That way less food is consumed, but mentally it still feels almost like a whole day off. In so doing, she was increasing her body weight less after each earned day (evening) off. If not taking a whole day off, an evening off is preferred over a morning or midday because you want to finish your day without limitations. Most people can mentally relax better this way.

The bottom line: if weight gain after a day off bothers you, but you still want your "pigging out" escape, take only an evening off and you will refresh your mind and reduce weight increase the next day.

Two consecutive and scheduled days off

When I dieted for certain bodybuilding shows, I sometimes took two consecutive days off every week, usually Friday and Saturday. Even though they were scheduled on a weekly basis, which I typically suggest to be wrong conceptually, they worked very well for me. I knew my body and accomplished my desired weight loss every time prior to days off. I earned my scheduled days off.

At the time I decided I would rather work like a "slave" Sunday through Thursday in order to reach my short-term fat loss goal, and therefore deserve two consecutive days off. I felt I needed two days off, because during the first day off I could mentally relax better knowing I had one more day to eat. The second day off I was not craving food as much as the first day, and it was easier to go back on the diet again. Often on a second day off I worked out even though I did not diet because I was physically stronger from eating the previous day and I could accomplish more intensive workouts.

The bottom line: adjust days off (and everything else) to your specific and unique physical and mental needs. Even if generally considered wrong, maybe you can adapt scheduled days off towards reaching your goal because you have the motivation and desire to do so.

Misuse of days off

During conditioning for a bodybuilding show, a younger colleague of mine decided to apply the idea of days off. Unfortunately, he disregarded everything except the part where I said, "Days off will not hurt your conditioning". In addition to too frequent days off, his diet and trainings were insufficient. After almost two months of failing to reduce fat deposits, I convinced him to stop taking days off, and stick with his fat loss regimen all the way to competition. That worked better for him.

The bottom line: days off are not for everyone. If they become too tempting, chances are you will start taking them too often.

Your body will follow your mind

One of my clients started experiencing serious mental crises because of her strict diet only three weeks before a fitness show. The quality of her trainings was significantly decreasing. In the middle of one training session I told her to stop exercising, go home and for the next three days do nothing but have fun and eat whatever, and as much as, she wanted. At first she thought I was kidding, but then she complied. Three days later, she was back completely mentally ready and focused. She finished her conditioning as expected and did very well at her show.

The bottom line: our mind is the limiting factor regarding fat loss, not our body. If you get your mind going in the right direction, your body will follow for sure. The body itself has no such sense of direction. In order to satisfy your mind and restore mental power and direction, sometimes radical but reasonable steps are needed.

A FEW USEFUL TIPS

Think about fat loss like a long distance you have to cross. It is your choice if you will cross it by walking slow and not taking a break until the end (i.e. not taking days off), or by alternating periods of walking or even running with periods of resting (i.e. taking days off).

Dieting for fat loss is stressful. Taking a day off is stepping away from the stress. The longer you step away from it, the harder it will be mentally to get back to it. In addition to the risk of gaining fat again, this is also a strong reason why it is not recommended to take more than three consecutive days off. Typically I suggest taking only one day off.

When on a day off, not all the excessive energy you have consumed in such a short time will get stored as fat. As an exaggerated example, if you consumed 35,000 excess calories on your day off, you will not store 10 pounds of fat that day. The body can only absorb so much in a given period of time, and the majority of that energy will just pass through the body without being used. Imagine an empty glass. Even if you spill a five-gallon bucket of water over that glass, most of the water will spill out, and the glass will retain only its usual amount. Similarly, no matter how much you over-eat in one, two or three earned days off, you cannot accumulate a noticeable amount of fat. Of course, if you consume excessive energy over a prolonged period of time, you will indeed store and gain fat noticeably, "one glass at a time". While the body will not use 100% of the energy offered by consumption, 100% of required energy for the body's life functions and daily work

> *The body will NOT use 100% of consumed energy. Much of it will just pass through the body.*

will have to be supplied from somewhere. No machine or organism can function without its baseline of energy. If you diet by numbers and consume fewer calories than your body needs, all the remaining calories will have to be supplied from previously stored energy (like fat deposits). In contrast, all the excessive energy from overeating will not be stored in fat.

After a longer period of fat loss, your stomach will temporarily shrink and you will not be able to consume the same amount of food as you did before the diet. This is a natural, limiting factor in the amount of food you eat during days off. You will notice it especially if you take only an evening off. In such a limited amount of time, your eyes will want to eat everything, but your body will be able to take in only a small fraction.

PERSONAL TRAINER

Contrary to some opinions, a good trainer helps much more than just by counting repetitions, adjusting seat height and picking up weights after clients. A good trainer will amplify your ability to achieve your goals safer, faster and easier. The trainer will also make the gym environment less intimidating by explaining what different exercises and machines do. In spite of all these good things, a trainer cannot lose fat for you. A trainer can point you in the right direction, but your fat loss success depends on your own efforts.

A TRAINER IS LIKE A TAXI DRIVER

Starting an exercise and diet program hoping to achieve a goal, but without knowing enough about it, is like trying to find an address in a foreign city without a map or anyone to help. Having an exercise or diet program is like finding that address with a map of the city. You will find it eventually, but probably not quickly or effectively. Having a good trainer is like using a good taxi driver. Even better than having a map, you will reach your destination in the most optimal way.

TRAINERS COME IN ALL VARIETIES

The concepts in this book are undeniable, but as I mentioned many times, the same goal can be achieved in countless ways. Every trainer has an individual style, and variety is welcome. Therefore, a trainer using different words or having a different presentation style than this book suggests does not make him or her a wrong choice, as long as he or she doesn't say something opposed to logic or the laws of nature. You should also not confuse a popular and sweet talking trainer with a really good and knowledgeable trainer. Those attributes are very different, though it is possible for someone to have both.

I will not try to describe everything that makes a good trainer, but following are some general ideas. In order to make a good choice, pay attention to someone's education, but even more so, their experience. The more knowledge and experience a trainer has related to your goal, the better. However, you do not necessarily need the best trainer. Most clients need only basic services (typically fat loss is one of them), and they will be just fine with a trainer with moderate knowledge and experience. A more knowledgeable and experienced trainer is certainly preferable for anybody, but there is no need to waste your time hoping for "perfection". Start with a good enough trainer now, rather than waiting for the perfect one to come along.

The trainer also has to show a high level of professional respect for the client, including genuine interest, strong initiative, and undivided attention. You do not want a trainer that is watching TV, bonding with his cellular phone, or talking to other people while supposedly training you.

> *Pick a trainer with a personality and style you like.*

Additionally, there are many good trainers out there, and with such a large selection, you should go for someone with a personality and style you like. That is almost equally as important as knowledge and experience. Pick someone around whom you will be comfortable during your sessions.

A GOOD TRAINER WILL READ YOU

When you start executing a specific training program, a good trainer will "read" you during the workout and adapt the program to your moment by moment needs. However, keep in mind, the trainer is not inside your body and does not feel everything you feel. The trainer can only navigate by what you say or by the signs you show while working out. Such signs are rhythm of breathing, display of strength and endurance, form of exercise, level of motivation, and so on. These signs reveal a lot, but not everything. Therefore, keep the trainer precisely informed about your current state. Do not hide information from your trainer. By pretending you can do more (or even less) than you actually can, for instance, you will just mislead the trainer and potentially harm yourself.

PIZZA NOT EGG WHITES

A good trainer must find ways to adapt training and nutrition to the client's capacities and reasonable comfort zones. For instance, one of the most efficient fat loss diets includes egg whites as a source of high quality protein. But in spite of its efficiency, not all clients will readily accept eating egg whites. It is irrelevant if egg whites are the best source of lean protein if a client will not eat them. In that case, the trainer must choose a lesser alternative that will still be good enough and acceptable for a client.

If a client eats a small pizza every day for lunch and does not want to change, it will be better if the trainer suggests eating only half of that pizza, rather than forcing a perfect diet that includes egg whites on him. The same thing goes for exercising. If the client hates squats, for instance, a trainer should suggest an alternative.

A friend of mine has a first-hand, successful experience of this type of adaptation. Her husband was a body builder and insisted on her using "perfect" fitness magazine diets, and fancy cutting-edge supplements in order for her to lose fat. This didn't produce any results because she absolutely rejected the idea of following such rigid programs. I told her she should not worry about so-called perfect diets, but instead she could create her own diet using any food that she likes, while of course eating less than she typically might. Months later she told me that she applied my advice, and designed her diet to include the previously "tabooed" bread, pasta, cheese, fruit, and even chocolate. Additionally, she made only minor adjustments to her lifestyle in order to become more active, not by going to the gym regularly as her husband had insisted, but simply by taking the stairs, and doing more of what she truly enjoyed, like gardening. She successfully lost all the weight she wanted, and divorced the guy a few years later.

While a trainer should be flexible in finding the best solutions towards achieving a client's goal, a trainer should also not stubbornly insist on changing a client's goal. If a client wants to lose 10 pounds of fat, and the trainer thinks the client should gain five pounds of muscle instead, the trainer can express an opinion, but must respect the client's final wishes. If a client's goals are too opposed to a trainer's convictions, the two individuals should probably not work together.

VOODOO FAT LOSS APPROACH

Occasionally I come across the following scenario when talking to people using trainers: a trainer may have accomplished very successful fat loss himself, and now, due to lack of experience, insist on his clients religiously following every step of his fat loss program. The following example is an exaggeration to make the point more clear.

A trainer might think that consuming shakes exclusively from a tall glass, not drinking water when the moon is full, and working out in a purple shirt worked for them in losing fat, and therefore that client must do the same. The fact is the trainer lost fat only because of energy deficit, not his or her voodoo approach to fat loss. Such approaches serve only the purpose of preoccupying the mind, and therefore make it easier to endure fat loss. Unfortunately, what works well for one person, won't necessarily work equally well for another.

If your trainer insists on you following his or her fat loss footsteps to the exact detail, know that you do not have to if it does not fit your preferences. The only thing you must do to lose fat is create energy deficit. How you are going to create that energy deficit and what voodoo approach you will use to preoccupy your mind is a very individual choice, and completely up to you.

DIE HARD APPROACH –
YOUR CHOICE, NOT NECESSITY

You may come across trainers that have a pretty extreme approach to training and nutrition. If you wish to become a professional athlete, you will have to put up with extreme conditioning, but for everyday life, that is not necessary. Desired results can be achieved in a very civilized, fairly comfortable way and you don't have to put up with a "survival of the fittest" conditioning approach.

A good example of a very extreme trainer is one colleague of mine. He himself was an internationally successful athlete, and definitely knew training and nutrition very well, no question about that. However, his training philosophy was horrifying. If you signed up for training sessions with him, you had the following choices: (1) die hard lifting, (2) drop dead starving, or his preferred option, (3) both. After a few weeks with him, his clients looked like prisoners from the Rambo II movie. Know that you do not have to accept this kind of conditioning. There are easier ways to your goal. However, some clients are fond of extreme programs, and, therefore, should go for it.

HOW MANY
TRAINING SESSIONS TO BUY

When deciding how many training sessions to buy, I suggest a conservative approach. Do not buy more than you can reasonably afford. A good trainer can teach you a lot even in just a few sessions. In addition to bringing in knowledge and experience, trainers are usually very helpful in maintaining a higher level of long term motivation necessary for success. They are like check points. When you meet with a trainer, you want to show them that you were dedicated to your goal and completed your "homework" since your last session. The trainer is someone to be accountable to, in a good way.

If you know enough about training and proper nutrition and have a goal oriented, very motivated personality, you do not necessarily need a trainer in order to reach your goal. Keep in mind, though, the risk of relying only on your own knowledge is that most people think they know much more than they really do. However, no matter how much you know, even if you

Your trainer is someone to be accountable to in a good way.

are the best athlete in the world, with all the knowledge and experience needed, you can still benefit from a good trainer. It is always beneficial to hear a second opinion, especially from an objective and knowledgeable person.

CHAPTER SIX

Reading nutritional information is just about as interesting as reading phone book listings. However, some listings are more crucial than others. This chapter won't make nutritional information any more interesting, but it will point out what's important and simplify it. It teaches you how to read nutritional labels, use tables of food contents, which foods to select for your diet, and how many meals to eat. In this chapter you will also receive step-by-step information on how to create meals and menus for your optimal fat loss program. If you are dieting by numbers and want to create the most effective program, this information is for you.

UNDERSTANDING NUTRITIONAL INFORMATION

Food you purchase most likely has a label with nutritional information on its packaging, but if it does not, you can usually find all necessary information in tables of food contents.

FOODS WITH A LABEL

If the food packaging has a nutritional label, it should at a minimum provide information about: total energy value, amounts of nutrients, and ingredients.

Nutrition Facts	Amount/Serving	% DV*	Amount/Serving	% DV*
Serving Size 1 bar (78g)	**Total Fat** 6g	**9%**	**Potassium** 90mg	**3%**
Calories 300	Sat Fat 3.5g	18%	**Total Carb** 38g	13%
Calories from Fat 50	Trans Fat 0g		Dietary Fiber 0g	0%
*Percent Daily Values (DV) are	**Cholesterol** 0mg	0%	Sugars 20mg	
based on a 2 000 calorie diet	**Sodium** 200mg	8%	**Protein** 23g	46%

Vitamin A 0% - Vitamin C 100% - Calcium 35% - Iron 40% - Vitamin E 100%
Thiamin 100% - Riboflavin 100% - Niacin 100% - Vitamin B6 100%
Folate 100% - Vitamin B12 100% - Biotin 100% - Pantothenic Acid 100%
Phosphorus 35% - Magnesium 30% - Zinc 35% - Copper 40% - Chromium 20%

Total energy value

Total energy value of the entire or partial product is the single, most important piece of information for fat loss. You do not have to worry about how many calories come from which nutrients (for example, calories from fat).

Calories may be expressed for a smaller amount of the product (for example, only one serving), and not for the whole package. Make sure

ENERGY DEFICIT IS THE ONLY TRUTH TO FAT LOSS.

you check for the quantity of product that the information refers to. Diet sweeteners like to say "Zero Calorie" (or "No Calorie") but that is not accurate. What they are saying by "Zero Calorie" is that you have less than one calorie per serving, but servings could be so small that they do not adequately represent the amount you will actually need to use. The amount you really need could include more servings, and that is not "Zero Calorie" any more. Regardless, diet sweeteners can be a great help during fat loss.

Please note, there is some controversial data around artificial sweeteners, so be sure to do your own research before including them in your diet.

The amounts of nutrients

The amounts of nutrients might be listed for the entire contents, or only partial contents. It is important to pay attention primarily to grams of protein. You want to consume a certain amount of protein per day since it is the major building material for the body, and the body cannot produce it sufficiently. High quality protein sources are different from low quality protein sources. You can check information about the protein quality source from the ingredients part of the label.

The grams of fat and carbohydrates in a product are irrelevant. Their relevance for fat loss is only the energy they provide, and that is reflected in the product's energy value. Grams of proteins are also reflected in the product's energy value.

Nutrition Facts	Amount/Serving		Amount/Serving	
	Total Fat 6g		**Potassium** 90mg	
	Sat Fat 3.5g		**Total Carb** 38g	
	Trans Fat 0g		Dietary Fiber 0g	
	Cholesterol 0mg		Sugars 20mg	
	Sodium 200mg		**Protein** 23g	

Other essentially unimportant information for fat loss is the percentages on the far right of the label. They represent how much of the daily required amount you have ingested of each nutrient by consuming that product. In our example, if you eat this energy bar you have consumed 23 grams of protein and that would be about 46% of the total required protein if you are on a diet of 2000 calories per day.

Nutrition Facts		% DV*		% DV*
		9%		3%
		18%		13%
				0%
*Percent Daily Values (DV) are		0%		
based on a 2 000 calorie diet		8%		46%

The ingredients

The ingredients used in the product should be listed in the order of their content, highest to lowest. For fat loss the ingredients are significant only for determining the quality of the protein you are consuming. You want to select products that have a higher content of high quality protein, like whey, milk and egg protein. Also, it is important to pay attention to the ingredients if you have a food allergy, intolerance or other medical condition requiring nutritional attention, but that is outside of this book's jurisdiction.

Calorie check for a nutritional label

We will break down the total energy value of the energy bar that was presented in the previous example into its three major components. According to the nutritional label, the total energy value of this bar is 300 calories, coming from the following energy-rich nutrients: 6 grams of fat, 38 grams of carbohydrates and 23 grams of protein. As a reminder, one gram of fat releases nine calories, and one gram of carbohydrate or protein releases four calories.

Fats 6 grams	54 calories	18 % of total energy
Carbohydrates 38 grams	152 calories	51 % of total energy
Proteins 23 grams	92 calories	31 % of total energy
Total energy	298 calories	100%

According to our calculations, there are 298 instead of 300 total calories. Such small differences are acceptable and happen often.

FOODS WITHOUT A LABEL

If the food does not come with a nutritional label you can still collect all the information you need. You should know the exact name of the product you are about to consume in addition to using tables of food contents and a food scale.

Tables of food contents

Tables of food contents are basically nutritional labels representing a wide variety of foods that have been collected together into one source. They can be found as independent publications, parts of other books, or on the Internet. Tables of food contents will usually provide plenty of nutritional information, more than you will need for your basic fat loss. However, sometimes the information they provide can be incomplete because it might be adjusted to fit various trendy fad diets, and not a reasonable fat loss program.

Choosing tables of food contents

First pick tables of food content that provide information on the energy values and protein content of different foods. Some tables will present only grams of carbohydrates or fats and their energy value. This is not necessary.

Next, I suggest you select tables that express values very precisely, preferably in grams rather than ounces only. For example, tables that list values for 100 grams of apple will be preferable to tables giving values for "an average size" apple. The exact specification of an average size apple is unknown; however, "100g of apple" is clear. Then you can use your food scale, measure your portion of apple, and very accurately determine its nutritional specifications.

Choose tables of food contents that are simple to use and small enough to carry with you. If you are away from home it is handy to have them with you. While on the road acquiring nutritional information from the Internet is practical also.

Using tables of food contents

When using tables, pay attention to the food's name, condition and quantity. For example, check if the data includes whether the food is raw, cooked, or peeled, and if it matches the quantity you are about to consume.

Following is an example of a simple table of food contents. I have included only basic foods most commonly used for fat loss dieting. Additionally, I have also included some energy rich foods to demonstrate how energy values can be drastically different between foods.

Foods are listed by their energy value and divided into two categories according to the quality of protein they provide.

Depending on the table you use, you may also encounter more detailed subcategories for each of the main foods, and entries for additional information like cholesterol, fiber, vitamins and minerals. Values presented in this table are approximate (page 166, 167).

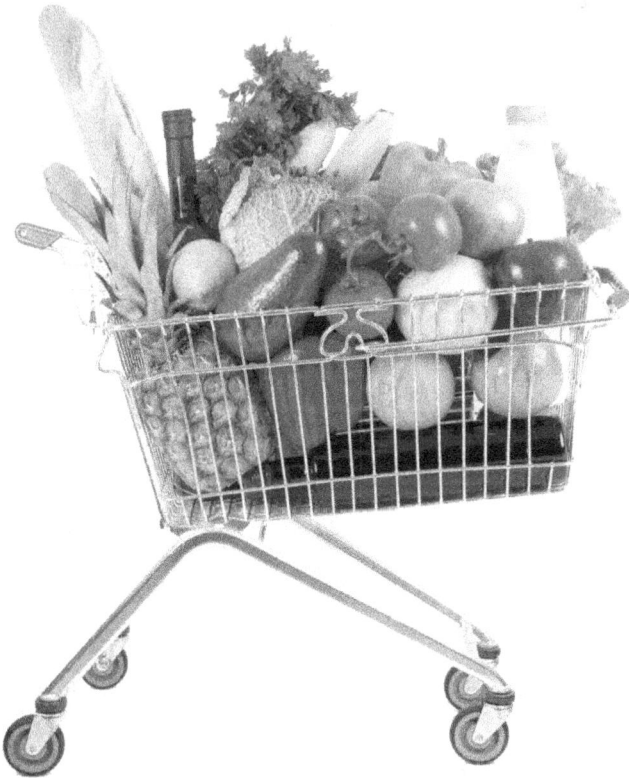

CATEGORY ONE Foods with *low* quality proteins ("incomplete" proteins)					
Food	Amount	Cal	Prot	Fat	Carb
Lettuce, raw	3.5 oz. (100g)	*11*	1.0g	0.2g	1.3g
Cucumber, raw	3.5 oz. (100g)	*12*	0.6g	0.2g	1.9g
Mushrooms, raw	3.5 oz. (100g)	*15*	2.7g	0.2g	0.6g
Tomato, raw	3.5 oz. (100g)	*18*	1.0g	0.2g	3.0g
Green pepper, raw	3.5 oz. (100g)	*20*	1.3g	0.3g	3.0g
Spinach, raw	3.5 oz. (100g)	*23*	2.1g	0.3g	3.0g
Cauliflower, raw	3.5 oz. (100g)	*25*	2.0g	0.1g	4.2g
Onion, raw	3.5 oz. (100g)	*28*	1.4g	0.2g	5.1g
Strawberries, raw	3.5 oz. (100g)	*29*	0.8g	0.4g	5.5g
Broccoli, raw	3.5 oz. (100g)	*34*	2.1g	0.4g	5.5g
Watermelon, raw	3.5 oz. (100g)	*38*	0.6g	0.2g	8.4g
Peach, raw	3.5 oz. (100g)	*44*	0.9g	0.3g	9.5g
Plum, raw	3.5 oz. (100g)	*46*	0.7g	0.3g	10.1g
Orange, raw	3.5 oz. (100g)	*47*	0.9g	0.1g	10.6g
Pineapple, raw	3.5 oz. (100g)	*48*	0.5g	0.1g	11.2g
Apple, raw	3.5 oz. (100g)	*52*	0.3g	0.4g	11.7g
Kiwi, raw	3.5 oz. (100g)	*61*	1.1g	0.5g	13.1g
Grapes, white, raw	3.5 oz. (100g)	*69*	0.7g	0.3g	15.9g
Fig, raw	3.5 oz. (100g)	*74*	0.7g	0.3g	17.2g
Potato, raw	3.5 oz. (100g)	*78*	2.0g	0.0g	17.6g
Banana, raw	3.5 oz. (100g)	*95*	1.2g	0.2g	22.0g
Ice cream (vanilla)	3.5 oz. (100g)	*201*	4.5g	10.2g	22.7g
Bread (white)	3.5 oz. (100g)	*240*	8.8g	0.9g	49.1g
Rice, white, dry (long grain)	½ cup (100g)	*360*	8.0g	0.9g	80.0g
Chocolate (milk)	3.5 oz. (100g)	*551*	8.9g	32.0g	57.0g

CATEGORY TWO Foods with *high* quality proteins ("complete" proteins)					
Food	Amount	Cal	Prot	Fat	Carb
Egg white (hen)	1 (25g)	*13*	*3.0g*	0.0g	0.2g
Whole egg (hen)	1 (63g)	*70*	*6.0g*	4.6g	1.0g
Cottage cheese (fat free)	3.5 oz. (100g)	*71*	*12.0g*	0.0g	5.7g
Tuna (in water)	3.5 oz. (100g)	*80*	*17.9g*	0.9g	0.0g
Tilapia	3.5 oz. (100g)	*91*	*17.7g*	2.2g	0.0g
Turkey breast	3.5 oz. (100g)	*93*	*14.2g*	4.0g	0.0g
Chicken breast	3.5 oz. (100g)	*98*	*19.6g*	2.2g	0.0g
Salmon	3.5 oz. (100g)	*146*	*25.9g*	4.7g	0.0g
Beef (rib-eye steak)	3.5 oz. (100g)	*259*	*18.7g*	20.5g	0.0g
Swiss cheese	3.5 oz. (100g)	*361*	*28.0g*	27.7g	0.0g
Water	Any	*0*	0.0g	0.0g	0.0g
Diet soda	1 can (355 mL)	*0*	0.0g	0.0g	0.0g
Milk (fat free)	1 cup (240mL)	*80*	*8.0g*	0.0g	12.0g

Food scale

Nutritional labels and tables of food contents provide nutritional facts for a particular amount of food, for example a serving size. Sometimes you will want to consume more or less than the serving size. In such cases, you can use a food scale to determine the difference between the size of your actual portion and the serving size specified on the label or in the table. When you determine the difference, adjust the nutritional information to fit your portion size.

Choosing a food scale

Pick a digital scale that expresses results in grams rather than only in ounces (most of them are that way). This suggestion has nothing to do with my European origin and preference for the metric system, but is because grams are smaller, more frequently used units when it comes to food.

The digital scale should have an accuracy of measuring as little as only one gram of food, and a maximum measuring capacity of at least 1000 grams (2.2 pounds). Most non-commercial food scales will have a high enough maximum measuring capacity but unless they are digital, they will usually not be accurate enough. It is also handy to have a small scale that is easy to transport if you travel.

Using a food scale

When weighing food, usually you should measure it before food preparation. After cooking, the values will likely change. For example, 100 grams of chicken breast will weigh a few grams less after cooking due to water loss. On the other hand, 100 grams of rice will weigh much more after cooking because of water absorption. When I prepare rice during my diet, I end up with about 400 boiled grams from the original 100 dry grams.

How to use tables and a food scale

We will assume, for example, you want to consume 50 grams of rice and intend to locate the necessary nutritional information to log it in your fat loss journal. Rice usually comes with a nutritional label on the package, but we will imagine it does not. These are the steps you would need to follow.

- Measure 50 grams of rice, dry right from the package.

- Look up the nutritional information for the exact name, condition and quantity of rice from your tables of food contents and log it into your journal.

- Start boiling the rice in water without adding any energy-rich substances (for example oil, sugar, and so on).

- After the rice is boiled, consume it without adding any energy-rich substances. If you do add oil or sweetener, the energy value will have to be adjusted to include additional substances.

We said that for a fat loss diet, the important nutritional information is total energy and grams of high quality protein. Considering the fact that rice is not a high quality protein source, you can disregard grams of protein and pay attention only to energy value. Therefore 50 grams of dry rice will have approximately 180 calories, and for your fat loss purpose that is all that needs to be recorded in your fat loss journal. However, if you have a food that provides a high quality protein (like an egg for example), then besides the energy value, you would also record grams of high quality protein, which you should count towards daily protein needs.

BE CONSISTENT
IN YOUR "MISTAKE"

The same food will sometimes have different nutritional values if you compare one source of information to another. For example, one table of food contents or nutritional label may say 100 grams of rice has 360 calories, and another could say it has 355 calories. Further, one package of eggs will say that each egg releases 70 calories, while some other source could state that one whole egg has 90 calories. The same variations could apply to all other nutritional information, not just a caloric value. Such differences appear often and you should not worry about them.

USE THE SAME SOURCE
AND LOG EVERYTHING

You should always use the same source of information for your foods, like the same table of food contents or the same nutritional label. Then, even if you are using one table or label that shows a bit less accurate information than another source, do not worry as long as you are consistent in your mistake. Use the same source of information and always log everything you consume in your fat loss journal. If you start frequently using various sources of information with noticeable differences in results, and you do not log everything, then you might create confusion.

If you log everything, but use a source of information that may be less accurate, you might think that you are consuming 1500 calories each day, when you are actually consuming 1600 calories. That is not going to harm your fat loss, as long as you always evaluate the practical efficiency of your diet; meaning, if you are not losing fat properly by current energy intake (calculated wrong or right), then adjust your diet and eat less energy. What counts is the fat loss result, not the exact precision of the number of calories. Naturally, you should try to find a source with as accurate nutritional information as possible.

STAY AWAY FROM RECIPES

During a fat loss diet, my suggestion is to generally stay away from complex food recipes. Pick about 10 simple foods that you like, learn their nutritional information, and stick with them. Select a few vegetables, grains, fruits, and high quality protein sources, eat them separately or mix them together, but keep it as simple as possible. Leave recipes for days off. That way your diet will be under better control.

If a complex food recipe comes with a nutritional label, then it can be a useful part of your fat loss diet. If nutritional information is not available, you cannot know its nutritional specifications unless you prepare it yourself.

When nutritional information is not available, and you have not prepared the food yourself, you can try to guess the nutritional specifications by breaking the food into its specific components. For example, if you are eating a hamburger, you can attempt to figure out the calories and protein for each component, such as the meat, bread, vegetables and so on. However, if you are hungry and the only food available has unknown nutritional specifications, simply eat a small amount in order to decrease the chance of consuming too much energy.

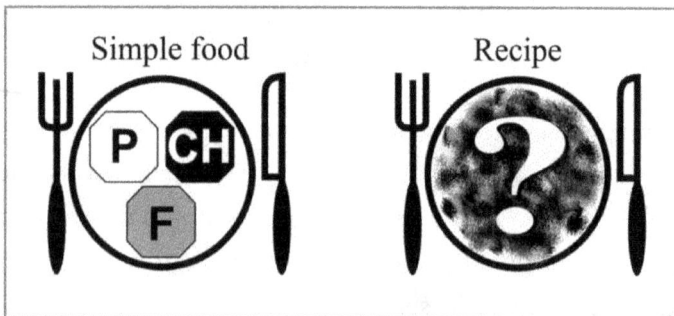

HIGHER IN PROTEIN,
LOWER IN CALORIES

When it comes to complex food recipes with unknown nutritional information, you can just assume there is no high quality protein. You risk consuming more protein by the end of the day, which is neither bad nor risky for your diet. However, by underestimating the overall energy of a food, you could over-consume your daily calories, and harm your fat loss progress. Within reason, you can consume more protein (more than recommended), but less calories (less than recommended), while dieting for fat loss.

PICK FOODS
WITH FEWER CALORIES

The idea behind picking foods with fewer calories is to be able to consume a greater amount of food with satisfactory taste and nutrient level, while keeping calorie intake low. We could say this is the main objective in shaping a fat loss menu.

To select foods with less energy, follow this basic guideline: try to find foods that have the smallest amount of energy per 100 grams (3.5 oz.) of weight. From these foods consider which ones you like and what nutrients they bring to your diet. Unfortunately, foods with very low energy usually do not taste very good, so you will probably have to incorporate foods richer in taste and energy into your diet too. During fat loss, balance between the amount and flavor of food is often required, and that can only be determined on an individual case-by-case basis.

NO PROTEIN,
FEWER CALORIES

Most vegetables and fruits will fit into this category, foods with no high quality protein and fewer calories. They should all have less than 100 calories per 100 grams of weight. They are low in energy, due to their high water content, as well as their lack of fat. When I diet, these foods provide me with a substantial volume of food so I feel full, but caloric intake is still low. In addition, some of them taste good and are a good source of dietary fiber.

WITH PROTEIN,
FEWER CALORIES

The most common foods with high quality protein and fewer calories are egg whites, some low fat milk products such as cottage cheese, chicken breast, turkey breast and tuna in water. These foods should have 125 or less calories per 100 grams of weight. They should also provide an average of 10-20 grams of high quality protein per 100 grams of weight. They are a bit higher in energy than the previously listed, no-protein foods because they usually contain less water and perhaps a few grams of fats. Additionally, some low-energy dietary products containing high quality protein are part of this group, and can come in very handy when forming your diet.

Some of the foods with fewer calories are listed in the table of food contents presented in the chapter "Understanding nutritional information", page 158-171.

WHOLE EGG VS. EGG WHITE

One example that illustrates the concept of saving energy while still consuming the required amount of nutrients is the difference between consuming a whole egg and egg whites.

If you eat a whole egg you will consume about 70 calories and six grams of high quality protein. However, if

> *Consume food rich in nutrients but poor in energy.*

you eat two egg whites, you will be much lower on energy (38%) compared to the energy of a whole egg, but your protein intake will be identical (100%). The major reason

for the difference is the fat content. Whole eggs have a significant amount of fat, while egg whites are basically fat free. The same thing applies to other types of food as well.

> *Think about food like you are taking medicine. Do not go for the flavor, but for the result you get.*

For your fat loss nutrition, pick foods that will give you more essential nutrients (primarily protein) for less energy.

That way if you occasionally wish to satisfy your cravings and consume energy-rich, tastier foods, you still have some space left before you reach your daily energy intake limit.

During fat loss, think about food like you do medicine. Do not choose food just for the flavor, but for the overall result. When you have a headache, do you search for a pill that looks and tastes good, or the one that will eliminate the headache?

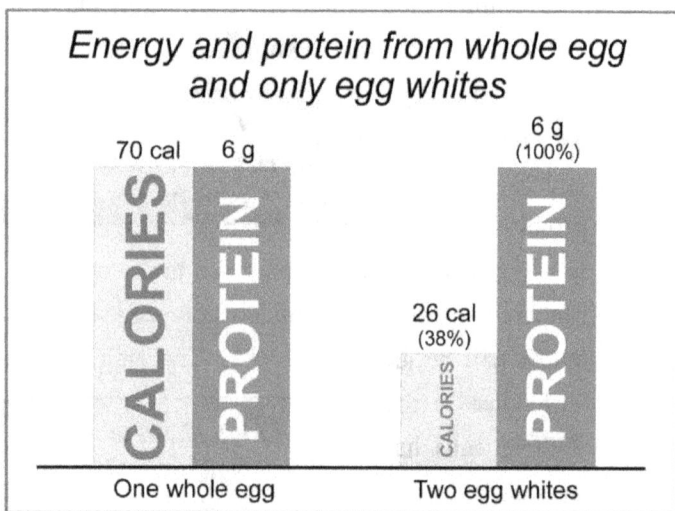

Energy and protein from whole egg and only egg whites

70 cal   6 g   — One whole egg (CALORIES / PROTEIN)

6 g (100%)   26 cal (38%)   — Two egg whites (CALORIES / PROTEIN)

EAT MORE
SMALL MEALS EACH DAY

It is best for fat loss to eat many small meals each day rather than one or two big meals. Naturally, the total energy of all meals consumed during the day (many small or one or two big) has to be about the same in either case, and within your targeted energy deficit.

By eating many small meals you will physically, but even more importantly, mentally handle a fat loss diet much better. If you have, for example, 10 very small meals each day, you will feel like you are eating all the time, even though the sum of the total energy could be very low. On the other hand, if you eat only once or twice each day, even larger meals, periods without eating will feel like they last forever. During these longer periods between meals, you are more likely to lose control over your diet and start overeating. In this book I refer to this as an accidental day off. This can be partially prevented by eating many smaller meals each day.

15 MEALS EACH DAY

If my clients are starting a serious fat loss program, I usually suggest they have five fairly balanced meals each day. Sometimes, the number of meals can go as high as 15 per day, especially if your targeted energy intake is high (for example, you are in energy deficit even while eating 2500 calories per day). However, no matter how many meals you have, you must remain in an overall energy deficit.

During fat loss you should not think about meals through conventional perception, for example, that a meal equals a steak with french-fries, apple pie and a beer. When losing fat anything you eat or drink that has energy is considered a meal, no matter how small it is. One meal can be comprised of only an apple, yogurt, protein drink, or glass of milk. Remember, try to incorporate at least a little high quality protein into every meal you consume.

> *By eating many small meals you will handle a fat loss diet better.*

If you are concerned about eating so often, do not worry. You will get used to it. At the very beginning of my bodybuilding career, a more experienced bodybuilder told me I would have to eat five times a day. That was such a shock to me. I thought, "How am I going to pay that much attention to food?" However, once I started, it became my normal routine, and after a while seemed like I had never done anything else.

EMERGENCY FOOD

During your diet it is very wise to always have some emergency food handy. It can be just about anything convenient to consume and is usually something you already eat during your fat loss program. It cannot require cooking or special preparation. My emergency foods are mostly apples, sometimes protein bars and occasionally bananas.

The emergency food is likely to be consumed when your daily schedule changes and you cannot get to the next meal as planned. For example, a meeting can take longer than expected or you can get stuck in traffic. Instead of starving until the delay is over, you can consume a small emergency meal. This prevents dips in blood sugar levels, and resultant food cravings.

PUTTING TOGETHER MEALS AND MENUS

People often ask me why I do not include fat loss menus in this book. They say it would be easier for them just to follow my predesigned menus, rather than create menus themselves. I have two main reasons for this decision.

First, there are way too many foods and menu options available. I could not possibly come even close to designing an optimal menu for each reader with his or her individual taste and nutritional needs. Second, if you are too lazy to form your own fat loss menu, you will also be too lazy to do what it takes to lose fat, even if I did include "divine fat loss menus" in this book.

The chapter "How strict is the diet?" (page 102-109) explains three basic ways you can diet for fat loss. If you decide to control your nutrition strictly and diet by numbers, in this chapter you will be shown how to formulate your meals and menus, step by step.

Choosing foods and drinks

To summarize, I suggest you choose 10 simple foods in order to have better control over your diet. Some of the foods must be sources of high quality protein. You also must pay attention to what you are drinking. Energy is energy, even when it comes from a liquid source. In my opinion it is best to consume drinks that contain no calories, such as water and diet drinks. You are better off consuming calories from food alone. If you drink a regular soda (12 fluid ounces), you will

> *You are better off consuming calories from food rather than drinks.*

consume significant energy (over 140 calories) but will not feel as full or as satisfied as if you had eaten the same number of calories from regular food, that you actually have to "chew and swallow". Some exceptions are food supplements. For instance, protein drinks can be very useful during your diet, and calories ingested by their consumption may be justified.

I like to consume diet sodas during my fat loss. After I drink one, I trick my mind and body into feeling more energetic and full in spite of consuming basically no calories. This has nothing to do with the possible presence of caffeine or other psychoactive stimulant drug, but with a sweet taste in my mouth and volume in my stomach. That trick does not last long, but it can be useful enough to successfully bridge periods between meals. As a reminder, there is some controversial data around artificial sweeteners, so be sure to do your own research before including into your diet drinks or foods that may contain them.

If I were to start a fat loss diet right now, these are the foods and drinks I would choose.

Foods	Drinks
Whole egg	Whey protein powder (high percentage)
Egg white	
Cottage cheese	Diet sodas
Yogurt	Water
Apple	
Tomato	
Rice	
Optional	
In addition, I would also consider taking supplements containing vitamins, minerals and dietary fiber.	

Now stop rolling your eyes. These choices are not the best choices for everyone's fat loss diet. They are just my choices, and I use them here only to explain the process of forming a fat loss meal and menu. Also, as my diet progresses, I could change these initial food choices. Throughout my career I have dieted with many different foods. However, some foods have always remained as staples in my fat loss diets, in particular, rice and egg whites.

Remember, there are more potentially effective fat loss menus and exercise programs out there than there are fingerprints on people who use them. In your food choices, you are limited only by your imagination. Using the lottery as an example, there are about 20 million possible combinations of 50 or so numbers. Imagine how many billions of food combinations are possible for your fat loss. In the lottery there is only one winning combination. By way of contrast in your fat loss there are endless winning combinations, so you do not have to put up with something you do not like. The one thing that never changes is the singular truth of fat loss, and that is energy deficit. Therefore, use the above only as an example, and choose your own food and drink.

Tally the grams of protein and calories for your chosen foods

The next step is to tally the exact number of grams of high quality protein and calories for your chosen foods and drinks. Try to list this information as uniformly as possible. For example, use the same amount of each food: I suggest 100 grams, which is about 3.5 ounces. Foods that are consumed as units, like one whole egg or one yogurt container, are exceptions. You can list their nutritional information referring to one unit. When you have your information uniformly listed like this, it will be easier to use it during your diet. It simplifies calculations significantly.

Following is the nutritional information for the foods and drinks of my choice.

Food/Drink	Amount	High quality protein (g)	Calories
Whole egg	1 (approx. 63 g)	6.0 g	70 cal
Egg white	1 (approx. 25 g)	3.0 g	13 cal
Cottage cheese (fat free)	3.5 oz. (100 g)	12.0 g	71 cal
Yogurt (fat free)	1 container, 6 oz. (170 g)	6.0 g	110 cal
Apple	3.5 oz. (100 g)	0.0 g	52 cal
Tomato	3.5 oz. (100 g)	0.0 g	18 cal
Rice (dry, before cooking)	½ cup (100 g)	0.0 g	360 cal
Whey protein powder (high percentage)	1 scoop (30 g)	20.0 g	120 cal
Diet sodas	1 can	0.0 g	0 cal
Water	Any	0.0 g	0 cal

Be sure to include information from additional sources such as energy from anything you used during food preparation or consumption. Also, supplements that you are using have to be included in the calculation in case they release energy.

As a reminder, grams of protein are listed only for foods that are sources of higher quality protein. Foods that contain lower quality protein, like rice, are only considered for their energy value.

Choose how much protein and calories you want to consume

The next step is to choose how many grams of high quality protein and calories you wish to consume during your fat loss program. For example, I decided that I want to consume about 125 grams of high quality protein and 2000 calories per day. No matter what numbers you settle on at the beginning, if those numbers do not produce satisfactory fat loss results, you will have to adjust them. Refer to "Proteins, energy-rich nutrients" (page 225-230) and "How Many Calories?" (page 116-125).

Decide how many meals you want to consume

I want to consume the 125 grams of protein and 2000 calories in five meals. I will have more substantial meals three times per day, as breakfast, lunch and dinner, and two smaller meals between. I will also try to consume high quality protein during most meals.

Divide calories and protein between meals

Since I am to consume 2000 calories during three larger and two smaller meals, I want to have about 500 calories during my breakfast, lunch and dinner (500 x 3 = 1500 calories), and about 150 calories during two smaller meals (150 x 2 = 300 calories). Over the course of these five meals I plan to consume 1800 calories. I will keep the remaining 200 calories available as needed. If any of the additional supplements, diet sweeteners or other food preparation items that I intend to consume will release energy, then they might be covered by those 200 calories. Alternatively, I will increase one of the meals if I feel especially hungry, or I will add a smaller meal (sixth meal), so I can bridge periods between my five scheduled meals. That sixth meal could represent consumption of an emergency food. However, if I do not need those 200 calories, I will not consume them. I will divide my planned 125 grams of protein somewhat evenly between meals.

Start forming your meals

This is how I would form my meals and menu according to the previous specifications and food choices (page 186).

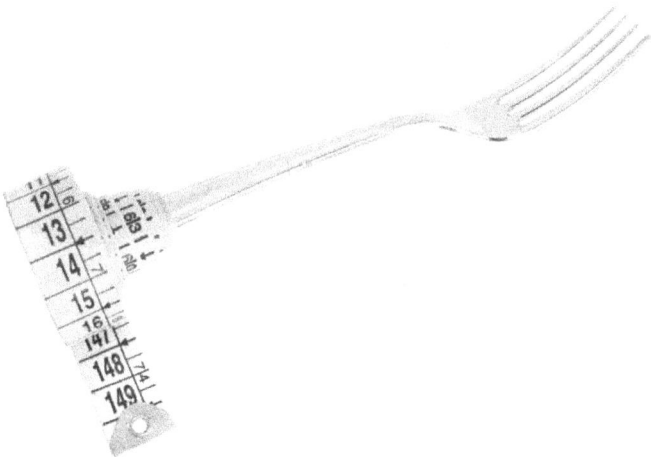

Food/Drink	Amount	High quality protein (g)	Calories
MEAL 1 (breakfast)			
Whole egg	3 (189 g)	18 g	210 cal
Egg white	3 (75 g)	9 g	39 cal
Tomato	6 oz. (170 g)	0 g	31 cal
Yogurt (fat free)	1 (170 g)	6 g	110 cal
Apple	one 8-9 oz. (250 g)	0 g	130 cal
Water or diet soda	Any	0 g	0 cal
	TOTAL for meal:	*33 g*	*520 cal*
MEAL 2 (morning snack)			
Yogurt (fat free)	1 (170 g)	6 g	110 cal
Apple	½ (125 g)	0 g	65 cal
Water or diet soda	Any	0 g	0 cal
	TOTAL for meal:	*6 g*	*175 cal*
MEAL 3 (lunch)			
Cottage cheese (fat free)	7 oz. (200 g)	24 g	142 cal
Rice	80 g	0 g	288 cal
Apple	½ (125 g)	0 g	65 cal
Water or diet soda	Any	0 g	0 cal
	TOTAL for meal:	*24 g*	*495 cal*
MEAL 4 (afternoon snack)			
Whey protein powder (mixed with water)	1 ½ scoops (45 g)	30 g	180 cal
	TOTAL for meal:	*30 g*	*180 cal*
MEAL 5 (dinner)			
Egg white	8 (200 g)	24 g	104 cal
Rice	50 g	0 g	180 cal
Yogurt (fat free)	1 (170 g)	6 g	110 cal
Apple	½ (125 g)	0 g	65 cal
Water or diet soda	Any	0 g	0 cal
	TOTAL for meal:	*30 g*	*459 cal*
	TOTAL FOR DAY:	123 g	1,829 cal

Reevaluation

I have planned to consume 125 grams of high quality protein and 1800 calories (plus reserve of 200 calories) from five meals during the day. After I formed my five meals, the total menu had 123 grams of high quality protein (2 grams under-planned) and an energy value of 1829 calories (29 calories over-

> *No need to nitpick.*
> *Be loyal*
> *to the general concept*
> *and you will lose fat.*

planned). I could have adjusted everything to the exact planned numbers, but there is no practical need for such precision, you are not building a Swiss watch. No real life diet will ever be, nor needs to be, 100% identical to its original plan. As long as you remain within a reasonable energy deficit, you will be fine.

Recommended flexibility

This example of food choices, meals and menu is presented only to give you an idea of how to put your own fat loss diet together. In reality, I usually do not attempt to form such a precise calculation of calories before every meal. I keep in mind my planned energy and protein daily intake, but try to save calories during the day and consume more as needed, such as after hard workouts for improved recovery, or in the evenings.

After a prolonged period of strict fat loss, it becomes especially hard to sleep on an empty stomach, so I prefer to consume a bit more food before I go to bed. In earlier stages of my bodybuilding career I promoted going to bed hungry, on an empty stomach. Now I have a different opinion. That does not mean that now I pig out in the evenings by any means. I consume my target energy, but distribute it differently. Even a few hundred additional calories during an evening meal will help you relax and sleep better. Fat loss is exhausting; you do not need to add lack of sleep to it.

Tear them up and start from scratch

Once you put your meals and menus together, you must try them out. If they don't fit you well enough, change them without hesitation. Change only the parts that you do not like, or if necessary, tear them up completely and start from scratch. However, be reasonable with your expectations. You can't avoid certain discomforts, but adjust your foods as much as you like while still paying attention to calorie and protein intake.

CHAPTER SEVEN

In the Wild West, we had the gold rush and gun fights. These days, we have the fat loss rush and fad diet fights. History repeats, go figure. Chapter Seven offers you insights into which dietary products you should and should not use during your fat loss fight. Some products will help you greatly. Others will only abuse your desire to lose fat, enabling Modern Day Snake Oil Salesmen to profit from it, and leaving you high and dry.

USEFUL DIETARY PRODUCTS AND SUPPLEMENTS

During any fat loss program, I am very much in favor of taking select dietary products and supplements. This is good nutritional support, but you should not overdo it. Always respect recommended dietary allowances or any specific directions for each product you use. Dietary products and supplements can be used for two basic reasons:

As a substitute for a whole meal (meal replacement products)

These products are usually in the form of a bar, drink, or powder. If you use a meal replacement product, especially on a regular basis, make sure that the product has the necessary nutrients for properly balanced nutrition. If you want to replace a meal once in a while, you do not need to be too concerned about nutritional balance. I believe that the body responds best if most of our meals are comprised of whole foods, rather than meal replacement products. Therefore, I suggest you do not over-consume them. Meal replacement products can come in especially handy as an emergency food.

Understand that fat loss meal replacement products can be very helpful in your fat loss program, but only if they replace conventional meals that are richer in energy, not if they are simply added to your regular diet. If you had a cheeseburger, French fries and apple pie, and after that also consumed a fat loss meal replacement product, don't hold your breath the next morning; your weight is not going down. Meal replacements are designed to provide you with a balanced, palatable meal, without too many calories. Like any other product, they

> *Do not over-consume dietary products and supplements and neglect whole foods.*

also contain no miracle ingredients that will burn your fat if you are not in energy deficit. If you simply add them to your usual daily nutrition, they will help you gain, rather than lose fat.

To supplement an improperly balanced meal (meal supplement products)

In this case, the product you are using should be primarily rich in the nutrients you are lacking in your meal. The most common examples are supplements containing vitamins and minerals. Vitamin and mineral supplements cannot properly replace an entire meal, but can only supplement it. Along with vitamin and mineral supplements, other popular products belonging in this category are high percentage protein, essential amino acids and dietary fiber.

I believe that vitamin and mineral supplements should be taken daily, even when not losing fat. There is no point in trying to meet your daily needs for vitamins and minerals through combining whole foods. That is just too difficult. Other supplements I recommend you seriously consider during your fat loss diet are those containing high quality protein and essential amino acids. However, unlike with vitamins and minerals, sufficient consumption of high quality protein is relatively easy to accomplish using conventional foods alone. You can also consume supplements providing dietary fiber, and essential fatty acids (see Appendix Two, "Nutrition", page 224-240).

FAT LOSS PRODUCTS

By the term "fat loss product", I am referring to a pill, capsule, supplement, drink, powder, lotion, "magic wand" or any other product that claims it will help you lose fat or body weight. When you read the rest of this chapter please do not think that I am saying that there is nothing out there that works for fat loss besides my book. On the contrary, there are many good fat loss programs. I will repeat what I said in the introduction. There are more potentially effective fat loss programs than there are fingerprints on people who use them. For them to be effective, they have to be done right. Therefore any program that promotes reduced energy intake and well balanced nutrition, along with proper physical activity in order to create an energy deficit will be an effective fat loss program. Any success story of such a fat loss program is also a success story for this book. That is because we are following the same and the only true fat loss principle - energy deficit. This being said, in the rest of the chapter I will focus on typical fat loss products and their empty promises.

I have been losing fat and manipulating my weight as a wrestler, bodybuilder and now recreational person for over 25 years, and during that time lost over 1500 pounds of my own body weight. If we add to it my clients and their weight loss under my guidance, the numbers are much greater. During all that time, I have never found one product that will make you lose fat and stay healthy by itself, or that will noticeably contribute to conventional fat loss produced by diet and exercise alone. However, people like fat loss products. When they ask me which ones to use, my answer is always, use none! Here is why:

First, often people use fat loss products knowing that they won't work, but wanting something to blame for their fat loss failure. They choose to be victims of imaginary unfortunate circumstances, rather than admit to their own laziness and then take responsibility for doing what it takes for successful fat loss.

Second, fatness is a natural occurrence, and fat loss should be achieved as naturally as possible. Seeking products to lose fat does nothing but add mystery and drama where they don't belong. I don't insist on "natural" everything, on the contrary! We just don't have anything "unnatural" that works well enough for fat loss.

Third, I am against fat loss products because in my experience they are fraudulent. They simply do not work. Here are some facts and thoughts you should consider:

- One hundred years ago we had far fewer fat people than today and also far fewer (if any) fat loss products.

- Today we have hundreds of fat loss products and many fat people are using them.

- The proof that people are using fat loss products is the existence (and growth) of the industry itself.

- Wouldn't it be logical to conclude that if fat loss products actually worked, anyone using them would not be fat anymore?

> *When people ask me what fat loss product to use, my answer is*
> *USE NONE!*
> *If any of them worked, fatness would already be a thing of the past.*

You draw your own conclusions, but this is what I think: if any of these fat loss products available today really worked, fatness would be long gone or at least rapidly decreasing, which is not the case. All these fat loss products did not appear because they worked, and were needed to "save the world" from fatness. Rather, they appeared to make money on the eternal human desire to achieve instant results with no effort.

> *Fat loss products are designed ONLY to make money on your desire to achieve results with no effort.*

Every day new products are coming out, their manufacturers' shouting aloud about their greatness and efficiency, but essentially they bring nothing new or improved, only different names disguising the same old short-term frauds and long-term disappointments.

CONVENIENT DISCLAIMER

Certain products also come with a convenient disclaimer, "This product works best in combination with a fat loss diet and exercise". Or sometimes they also give you a fat loss diet and exercise program you should follow while using their product. What a manipulation that is. Of course their product "works" best in combination with diet and exercise. Diet and exercise alone will do the job. Fat loss products will just take the credit for the success. However, if success does not come, then blame it on insufficient diet and exercise.

> *Manufacturers of fat loss products love to TAKE THE CREDIT for fat loss achieved by diet and exercise alone. But they NEVER ADMIT that their products are essentially worthless.*

Make no mistake, some products will dehydrate you, or clean out your digestive system and, therefore, drop your body weight significantly. This is not fat loss. These are only temporary changes to your body weight, and some are unhealthy. For example, when I competed, during the last six days before each competition, I used to drop 15-20 pounds. That was not due to fat loss at all, but only water manipulation. Fat loss happened gradually in the previous two to four months of dieting and exercising.

You must also know there are substances which will drug you out of hunger, appetite, fatigue, sleep, pain or a clear mind. Can you lose fat and drop your body weight by using them? Yes you can, but it is very unhealthy and the aesthetic results are usually unsatisfactory. Using such substances to lose fat will produce a similar result to that shown on a popular image used against smoking: "Smoking will make you lean" printed on the picture of a skeleton.

LET THE PLACEBO
DO THE WORK

Some people are prone to achieving a placebo effect. If you are one of them, go for it. Then, any product, even plain water, will "help" you, and you should use all the help you can get. Thinking a fat loss product will make a difference, you will start dieting and exercising more, and due to that lose fat. Again, I don't know even one person who has demonstrated fat loss success due to fat loss products alone. However, many have initially sworn on the greatness of some product they were using. Yet in this bottom line world, their physique did not change for the better.

ASTONISHING 3.86%

Most fat loss products have (or at least should have) clinical support for their effectiveness, but demonstration of their "field" effectiveness has proven practically insignificant. Among countless other examples, I recently heard a company brag about achieving 3.86% better fat loss in individuals taking their product compared to the control group (the people who didn't take the product for the research study). That's so remarkable. If those results are true, that means from one hundred pounds of lost fat, the contribution of the fat loss product is an astonishing 3.86 pounds. This is like driving a sleek, red sports car 150 mph, and then folding in the outside mirrors, hoping you will go faster. Diet and exercise will get you to 150 mph, whereas folding the mirrors is the contribution you could possibly expect from fat loss products.

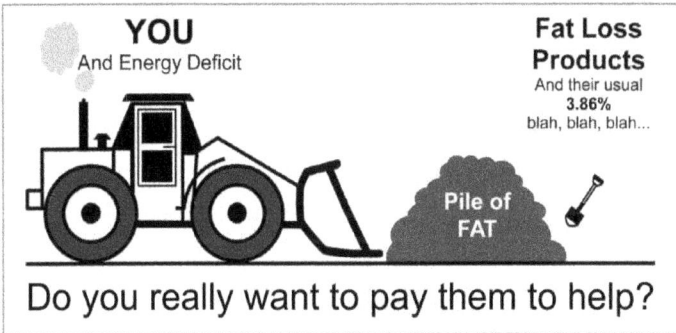

YOU
And Energy Deficit

Fat Loss Products
And their usual
3.86%
blah, blah, blah...

Pile of FAT

Do you really want to pay them to help?

ROCK SOLID OBJECTIVITY

In December 2011 I almost choked in Denver, not due to the "evil contents" of my fast food meal, but rather from an arrogant lie and manipulation I was hearing on the radio. They were seeking research candidates for their brand new, revolutionary, scientific breakthrough fat loss product.

The fact that they already knew their product was a huge breakthrough without having completed the research yet didn't shock me much. What did shock me was the criteria for candidates to qualify for their research: each candidate had to lose a minimum of 10 pounds in order to qualify for using the product.

If it were truly objective research, they would first give you their fat loss product, and then see how much fat you lost. In this devious approach, they insist on you losing 10 pounds, regardless of how you do it, so they can use your results to brag about the success of their product. Translation: their product doesn't work, and they need "doctored" results to uphold the illusion of their "revolutionary" product. What a scam!

In this country with laws and regulations about how often you are allowed to change your underwear, there aren't laws against schemes like this. Something is seriously wrong with a system that allows these clowns to walk free anywhere but within heavily guarded prison yards. Al Capone and all the other notorious criminals combined together did not pilfer as much money as these people do using their lies and manipulations.

TEST THE FAT LOSS PRODUCT

Even though the complete ineffectiveness of these products is so obvious, people keep looking skyward, teary-eyed, hoping for the "miracle pill" that will contribute to their success. Let me ask you honestly: do you really want to invest your hopes, money, and time delaying your own efforts while another charlatan delivers yet another deception that will supposedly help you lose 3.86% more fat? Stop staring at the sky, snap out of it and come back to Earth! Roll up your sleeves, and get to work on the real task at hand.

However, if even after these arguments, you still are seriously curious about the effectiveness of some fat loss product, go ahead and try it out. Start using the product of your choice, but change absolutely nothing else in your exercise, diet or lifestyle. If you did not exercise before, do not start. Do not eat any less or different food than before. After a while, see how much fat you have really lost.

IT MUST LEAVE YOU
FAT FREE

This experiment will not provide relevant data if you already are losing fat successfully through diet and exercise. It will be impossible to determine if the fat loss product contributed or not. You will obtain the most accurate conclusion if your body fat (body weight) remains stable for a longer period of time, such as six months. Then, if a fat loss product works, you should start losing fat gradually and constantly. But, again, change nothing else in your lifestyle! Daily and even weekly changes in body weight are not relevant, as these changes happen all the time, even without a fat loss product, training program or diet. If the product is really working, continuous fat loss will be evident as long as you are using the product. If you don't stop using it, all fat from your body should eventually be gone. If the fat loss product eliminates fat because it is genuinely effective, why would fat loss slow down or stop while you are still taking it?

Remember, if you are on a real fat loss program, with diet and exercise, there is no end to fat loss until you stop achieving an energy deficit and start consuming equal or greater energy than your body spends. Only then you will respectively either stop losing fat or gain fat again.

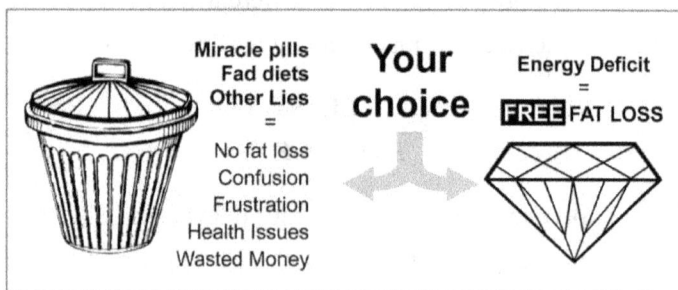

POWERFUL TOOL

Energy deficit is an amazingly powerful tool, and it can turn into a weapon if you push it too far. History teaches us about countless crimes and human suffering, such as Nazi prisoner-of-war camps. Together with other horrors, those people were exposed to severe starvation and hard manual labor resulting in gross energy deficit. None of these people were fat. No hormonal imbalance? No slow metabolism?

This dramatic example teaches us not to question whether energy deficit is the truth of fat loss. It commands us not to even compare it to other commercialized fat loss solutions, more aptly named, commercialized fat loss pollutions.

MORE FAT LOSS FRAUDS

There isn't much benefit to be found in fat loss products. My usual motto, "If I have nothing good to say, I say nothing at all", just doesn't apply. With so much pollution everywhere around us on the subject of fat loss, the truth, regardless of how it might sound, must be told.

In the same way, I must say that nearly everything I have mentioned so far about fat loss products applies to all the "easy", "instant" and "miracle" methods for losing fat. Such frauds can be referred to as fat loss supplements, medications or treatments, fashionable or fad diets, revolutionary training techniques and exercise machines, and so on.

Late-night television mercenaries describe their merchandise with words like, "never seen before", "life changing results", "clinically proven product", "scientific breakthrough", "the latest research" or other dramatic phrases. They will bring some all-knowing "hired gun MD" to add a medical spin to attempt to paralyze your objective thinking and convince you to buy their latest product. After all, you wouldn't dare question the knowledge and intentions of our knights in shining armor in the medical field. Additionally, they will likely use a "money back guarantee" or other, similar sales gimmick and manipulation to dupe you.

The bottom line is: no matter how convincing fat loss frauds are, nothing will make you lose fat to your satisfaction except energy deficit. That is the law of nature. The only way someone else but you can make you lose fat is if he or she locks you in a prison cell and underfeeds you until you are lean.

I suggest this simple practice. Every time you think about buying a fat loss product, reduce the size of your meal portions, walk around the block, and take half the money that you intended to spend and donate it to the charity of your choice (my money goes to animals). That will certainly deliver much better results for everyone.

MAKING A WEIGHT LOSS POINT

There are many cases when someone's radical weight loss is used as an advertisement for fat loss products or dieting methods. Such fat loss successes are commonly presented by dramatic before and after photos. We also come across contests on TV, in magazines, or other places, where people compete in losing weight under a deadline. All these results should be taken with serious reservations. The following is one of many possible reasons why such results should not be taken at face value.

When someone wants to prove how much body weight can be lost over a given time period, the process can be artificially manipulated as described in these three stages.

Stage one

At the beginning, a person can consume large amounts of food and liquid (and avoid going to the bathroom) to be as heavy as possible at the initial body weight measuring. This initial weighing represents the official beginning of the weight loss contest. Because of all that food and liquid artificially held in the body (not because of real fatness), body weight will be much greater than normal and the body will look overly bloated. These artificially-gained pounds will easily disappear a few days after the initial weighing during the process I call in this book, "initial quantum weight drop", but at a more exaggerated pace than what normally happens. That will deliver the first misleading evidence of rapid weight loss that has nothing to do with real fat loss.

Stage two

After this initial body weight measuring, the person will usually start an aggressive fat loss program. During this time, the objective is to reduce fat deposits as fast as possible. This is when real fat loss is occurring, and it will last until nearly the end of the contest. Compared to the initial quantum weight drop, this stage of real fat loss will reveal slower results in weight reduction. Better results will be achieved if the duration of the contest is longer, because actual fat loss is a slow process. This stage is not "bad" or "harmful" if not executed too strictly or under too much pressure to attain results in an unreasonably short time.

Stage three

Then, a few days before the final weighing, which represents the official end of the weight loss contest, the person can drastically reduce the amount of food and drink (consuming just enough to survive). By doing so, they will forcefully drop body weight again. In other words, before the final weighing, the person does almost the exact opposite sequence of actions than before the initial weighing. In addition, physical exercise can be applied aggressively to forcefully dehydrate the body and lower its weight. During the last few days sodium-rich food can also be avoided for more successful release of water. In more extreme cases, certain medications can be taken to empty the digestive system and force dehydration. The result is another sudden weight loss before the final weighing. This represents the second misleading evidence of rapid weight loss, and also has nothing to do with the real fat loss that happened during stage two.

By using the procedure described in the previous three stages, one can easily lose 20 or more pounds in one month. But out of those 20 lost pounds, maybe only 10 are from real fat loss. The other 10 are due to forceful retention of food and water before the initial weighing, and then forceful release before the final weighing.

Such a process is unhealthy and does not represent the right way to lose fat or reduce your body weight. If you wish to cause positive change to your body, lose fat, develop muscle, and improve conditioning, then you must be reasonable in your expectations and gradual in execution of the process.

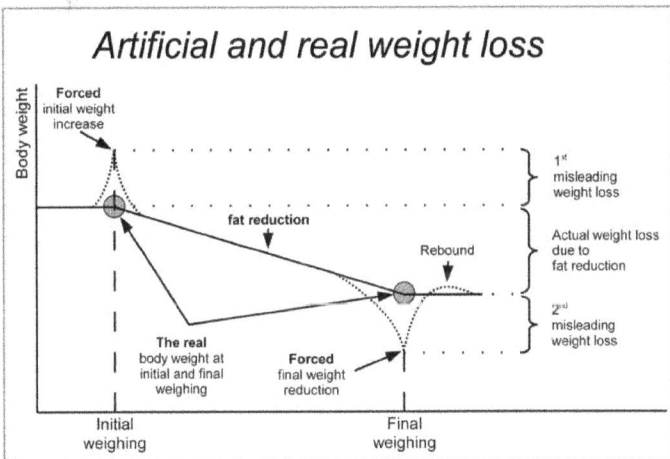

Artificial and real weight loss

THE AXIOM OF SUCCESS

No matter how hard you may try to blame genetics, hormonal imbalance, life circumstances, or other situations on your excess fat, what makes you fat is not the body's "wrong wiring" or the opening up of a new fast food restaurant in your neighborhood. What makes you fat is a lack of temperance. No matter how many trainers you hire, diets you try, products you consume, books you read, or therapists you see, in the end it is up to your power of will to finish the job and lose fat. Your fat loss (or gain) will come exclusively from within yourself, not from the environment that surrounds you. It is as simple as that. The sooner you accept it, the sooner you will lose fat or make peace with reality.

The axiom of any success in life, including fat loss, is discipline. If you have none, don't worry about losing fat, you will not succeed. On the other hand, if you find discipline to be a familiar and welcome aspect of life, I assure you fat loss will be another successful journey for you.

CHAPTER EIGHT

Chapter Eight is the final writing on the wall. Thou shalt not stay fat obeying these eight chapters. The following story will assure you of the certain effectiveness and wide applicability of the fat loss methods presented in this book. Consider, if this book were kept on the same shelf as Webster's Dictionary, the word "fat" would evaporate from its pages.

ASTRA'S FAT LOSS

This is a little story that describes well how losing fat by numbers and facts will be successful even under peculiar circumstances. Astra is my "cutie doggie girl"; she is Maltese, 13 years old, and has a heart condition. She used to be noticeably overweight. After the vet told me that her heart condition had gotten worse, we decided it would be beneficial for her to lose weight. The vet suggested certain brands of diet dog food, and gave me the usual amount of calories per pound that dogs need to maintain their body weight. That was helpful, but unfortunately she did not lose weight as expected, so I decided to utilize a more detailed approach.

I was very motivated but, at the same time, intensely worried about the task ahead of me. She is so much smaller than me and my human clients, so I couldn't apply my usual valid guess work regarding proper calorie intake for fat loss. Also, the fact that she could not express herself explicitly in a way I could completely understand about her fat loss experience was very concerning. I did not want to overdo it, but the result needed to be achieved quickly.

After significant consideration, I decided to carefully use on her the same approach I would use on myself. I picked about six different foods, pulled out my digital food scale, tables of food contents, and fat loss journal. I took her initial body weight and circumference measurements on four body parts, and started her diet with about three balanced meals per day. It took me about three weeks to figure out what calorie intake worked for her, but once I got it, it was just a question of precise execution. Periodically, I had to reduce her calorie intake to assure continuous weight loss. It was a bit of a challenge feeding the other three dogs their usual nutrition and keeping her on a strictly controlled fat loss diet, but with good organization it was successful.

Generally, I kept her on a strict diet Saturday through Thursday, and then Friday morning we would go to the vet's clinic to check her body weight. You remember the principles: always the same scale, on an empty stomach, at the same time of day, and so on. If she had lost weight since the previous Friday, or even if she had stayed the same (but no more than two weeks in a row), I gave her, along with the other dogs, a day off. A day off usually included a rotisserie chicken or smoked turkey legs, treats and other tasty snacks. Regarding exercise, I did not want to expose her to too much physical stress, considering her heart condition, so we went for moderate walks three to five days a week in the park nearby, and the rest of the time she had her back yard to play in and chase squirrels.

To summarize, at the beginning she was almost 13 pounds, had difficulty moving, and was panting nearly all the time. At the end of the diet, she was 8.8 pounds, very physically active, full of life, and hardly panting at all. At some circumference measurements she lost over four inches. Considering how much smaller she is compared to me, her result of losing four pounds is like me losing over 100 pounds.

I didn't write this chapter to discuss the love I have for my dog, nor to interest you in her health, but rather to show you that the methods described in this book are vastly applicable and effective. I used on her exactly what I use on myself, on my clients, and what I suggest you use in order to lose fat.

FAT LOSS CHECKLIST

Here is a checklist to remind you of the key things to do and consider before, during and after your fat loss.

Decision and preparation

1. *Reality check* – Decide if you really want to lose fat, and if you are willing to work for it almost every day. If you are not sure that you want to do it, don't even start. Start when you are truly ready.

2. *Determine your goal* – After you decide you are going to lose fat, set a realistic and meaningful goal, and give yourself reasonable time to reach it. Write down your goal and look at it daily.

3. *Check your health* – Before you take any action, check with your physician to see if your goal and intentions on reaching it are safe for your health. Also, ask how often you will need to come in for checkups.

4. *Get your journal, tables and scale* – If you want to diet by numbers, you will need a fat loss journal, tables of food contents and a digital food scale. Have them ready before you start your diet.

5. *Select your diet* – Pick, or better yet, design your own fat loss nutritional program, including foods you will eat during your diet. Principles from this book will provide you with clear guidelines in establishing the process.

6. *Nutritional information* – Gather needed nutritional information for each food that you will consume during

your fat loss (that is, grams of high quality protein and energy value).

7. *Determine your protein and calorie intake* – Establish your initial daily protein and energy intake for fat loss. Remember, the only thing that will make you lose fat is energy deficit.

8. *Form your meals and menus* – Compose meals and menus from foods you will eat during your diet, and pay attention to the grams of protein and number of calories.

9. *Select your physical activity* – Pick exercises that you are capable of and willing to perform during your fat loss.

10. *Go shopping* – Have all selected foods on hand before you start your diet. If required, also purchase needed supplies for your planned physical activity (for example, sneakers, clothing, ball, racket, bicycle, and so on).

11. *Record your initial condition* – Take your initial body measurements. I recommend recording your body weight, and circumference measurements. If possible, measure your body fat percentage, too.

12. *Take pictures* – Use before, during, and after photos to track progress. Make sure they are all taken under the same or very comparable conditions.

Execution

13. *Start your diet and keep it simple* – Consume your selected foods and apply your chosen physical exercise. Stay within a reasonable energy deficit daily; do not exaggerate by starving or over training yourself.

14. *Use a fat loss journal* – Record your information each day. Remember, it is most effective to diet by numbers and facts, not by feelings and guessing.

15. *Keep your mind in check* – Take it one day at a time. Try to preoccupy your mind with things other than food limitations and fat loss.

16. *Endure the first two weeks* – In the beginning fat loss can feel overwhelming, but it usually gets easier after the first two weeks.

17. *Work on smaller goals* – Create and stay focused on smaller, transitional goals, rather than the bigger final goal. Enjoy and regenerate your motivation by reaching every transitional success, however small.

18. *Consider your earned days off* – Are you taking enough? Too many?

19. *Keep checking your progress* – Take periodic measurements and pictures, check your fat loss journal, and determine if your progress is satisfactory or if you need to adjust your fat loss program.

20. *Recheck your health* – Periodically recheck your health at least as often as recommended by your physician.

21. *Keep doing what works* – If you are happy with your progress, keep doing what you're doing. Don't fix what is not broken. If you are not happy with your progress, then adjust your fat loss program.

22. *Watch out* – Stay away from any and all fat loss products, or programs that promise fast and easy success. The only thing that will make you lose fat is energy deficit, earned by your discipline and effort. Everything else is only clutter that confuses you.

Maintenance

23. *Keep the fat off* – After you have reached your goal, maintain a proper diet and continue physical activity. If you neglect a positive lifestyle, you will get fat again.

24. *Help your fellow man* – If this book was useful for your fat loss and you have friends who want to lose fat, tell them to buy a copy. Help them lose fat, and help me pay my bills.

APPENDIX ONE

If you expect this chapter to be an infomercial, delivered by a hysterical trainer wearing tights and a muscle shirt on a fat-free spray tanned body, psyching you up to get six pack abs before summer, you're reading the wrong book.

Appendix One illuminates the elementary things you need to know about exercise. It will explain two basic types of physical activities, and how they relate to your fat loss. You can use this knowledge to accelerate achieving your goal through structured physical activity or your everyday physical labor. Now drop and give me twenty.

EXERCISE

Fat loss physical activities can be divided in two basic categories:

- Aerobic physical activities
- Anaerobic physical activities

AEROBIC PHYSICAL ACTIVITIES

Aerobic physical activities (also known as cardio training in the context of fat loss) are all types of physical activities that are done with low intensity but high volume. Also, the movement must involve using 15% or more of a body's total muscle mass. For example, running with a slow speed of five miles per hour for 30 minutes is a typical aerobic activity. In this case, speed represents the intensity and time represents the volume of the physical activity. But running itself can also be anaerobic activity if done fast and short. For example, sprinting at the speed of 20 miles per hour for only 10 seconds is typical anaerobic activity because its intensity is high but volume is low. Therefore, it is not what activity you use, but how you use it.

Some physical activities are more suitable for aerobic training than others. Typical activities that are used for aerobic training are walking, running, riding a bike, rowing, swimming, and so forth. In fitness centers, aerobic training is commonly performed on cardio machines, including treadmills, stair climbers, elliptical machines, stationary bikes and rowing machines. However, for cardio machines to noticeably contribute to your fat loss, they have to be utilized for an extended period of time. Maintain exercise for 15 minutes or longer, if your health and physical condition permit. Typical fitness classes are also considered aerobic activities.

Aerobic exercise and burning fat

Aerobic activities are important for accelerated fat loss. When maintained for extended time periods, they burn a lot of energy. That energy can come either from current consumption of food and drink, or from previously stored energy, for example, fat deposits. If you adjust your energy intake below the body's needs, and use aerobic activity to increase the energy deficit even more, fat loss will be faster.

In addition to amplifying the fat burning process, aerobic activities are very beneficial for the health and function of the cardio respiratory system, and they help you to handle stress more efficiently. However, for the most part, they are not sufficient for maintaining and developing muscle tissue. For that you have to use proper resistance training. If you don't, there is a greater chance you will lose a noticeable amount of muscle tissue during your fat loss program. That is, if fat loss is accomplished only with diet, or with diet in combination with aerobic exercise alone.

How to apply aerobic exercise

If not problematic for your health and well-being, generally the longer you maintain aerobic activity, the better it is for your fat loss. The more time you spend exercising (physically working or moving), the longer your energy expenditure will be on a higher level. However, while exercising for fat loss, you generally should not apply too intensive of an aerobic workout that will increase your heart rate too much. During higher intensity physical exercise the body will use fat less efficiently and resort more to burning carbohydrates to satisfy its energy needs. Use lower intensity aerobic exercise, and you will exercise longer and also burn fat more efficiently. But if you like to blast it on "high intensity", go for it. You will still burn energy and fat, but you will probably not be able to exercise as long as you would with lower intensity.

To find out what a good heart rate is for you in order to burn fat the most efficiently, check the Internet, books, magazines and any cardio machine. Charts of optimal heart rate for fat loss, or other fitness goals are everywhere. For fat loss it is commonly recommended to stay in the zone of 55-65% of your maximum heart rate. The maximum heart rate is calculated by subtracting your age from 220. For example, if you are 40 years old, your maximum heart rate is 180 beats per minute. To be in the most efficient fat burning zone, you should keep your heart rate between 100 and 115 beats per minute (which is about 55-65% of 180).

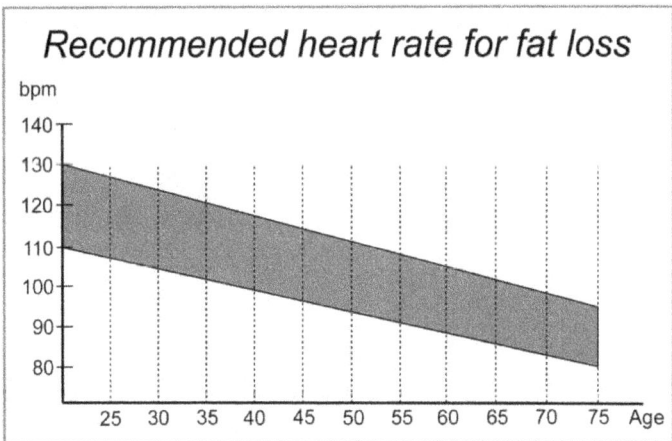

Recommended heart rate for fat loss

As an alternative to reading charts and checking your heart rate, you can navigate more generally by being aware of your breathing. If you are walking on a treadmill, for example, make sure you are capable of talking without getting too short of breath. You should be able to speak sentences without big breaks to catch your breath. If your speech is obviously broken, you are probably exercising too hard and should slow down a bit. Do not walk too slow either; your heart rate and breathing should be increased noticeably.

Do aerobic after resistance exercise

As a general rule for fat loss, when utilizing aerobic and resistance exercise in the same training, do resistance exercise first. A smaller period of aerobic exercise (5-10 minutes) can be done at the beginning, as a warm up, but the majority of aerobic exercise (for example, 30 or more minutes) should be completed after.

If you opt to do your aerobic exercise first, you could get too tired for proper execution of resistance exercise. Resistance exercise requires high intensity performance, plenty of motivation and determination. Therefore, it is optimally performed first, while you are still fresh and energetic. On the other hand, resistance training will not harm your aerobic activity because it can be performed on "auto pilot", requiring much less will power.

ANAEROBIC
PHYSICAL ACTIVITIES

Anaerobic physical activities have high intensity but low volume. They are significantly more intensive but individually much shorter lasting than aerobic activities. Typical examples of anaerobic activities are sprinting, jumping, throwing, and so on. In the context of fat loss, the most important anaerobic physical activity is resistance training, meaning exercising with free weights and resistance machines.

Resistance training saves muscles

Ideally, proper resistance training should produce progress in muscle strength, power and endurance, muscle mass and so forth. However, during fat loss the number one role of resistance training is to prevent or slow down loss of muscle characteristics.

It is possible that resistance training could cause muscle progress during fat loss. If you have never used resistance training before, and start using it for the first time at the beginning of your diet (or when your diet is not very strict), your muscles could progress a bit, in spite of energy deficit. During time your muscles could "wake up", and improve their strength, power, endurance or even size. Nevertheless, such progress is rare and will be limited and short lasting, because for proper muscle development you need enough energy and nutrients, while fat loss implies energy deficit and limited nutritional resources.

Overall, even if you use proper resistance training twice a day every day during your fat loss, it is likely you will still lose a certain amount of muscle tissue. The stricter your diet is, and the lower you wish to drop your body fat percentage, the greater your losses are going to be. With proper resistance training you can merely reduce this negative trend.

Because of their intensive but short nature, anaerobic activities are not the greatest energy spenders. They will absolutely contribute to overall energy expenditure, but not as much as extended aerobic activities. You may have heard that during the period of rest following resistance training, you will burn more energy than during the period of rest following aerobic training. Regardless, the best fat loss results will be achieved by a combination of diet, cardio and resistance exercise.

If for some reason you wish to choose only one type of physical exercise (either cardio or resistance training), choose resistance training. The resistance training will likely expend less energy, but will still spend noticeable energy while maintaining muscle mass. On the other hand, cardio will only expend energy and will not maintain muscle mass.

You can also adapt resistance training to have more aerobic characteristics. To do so, apply various resistance exercises in quick succession and without much rest between sets. Or while resting between sets you can add in a short period of cardio activity, like walking on a treadmill for a minute or two.

Muscle reaction to training

Muscle reaction to training can be explained simply as follows. If muscles are exposed to a new, higher than usual physical stress, they will tend to improve their characteristics to try to respond to the new demand. Improvement of their characteristics equals muscle progress. If muscles are exposed to the same physical stress over and over, they will maintain their current characteristics. However, if the level of physical stress is reduced from what muscles are used to, they will start losing their characteristics.

Depending on the structure of the applied physical stress, muscles will develop specific characteristics needed to satisfy the imposed demand. If you progressively lift heavier weights, muscle strength will increase. If you progressively lift more repetitions, muscle endurance will increase. If you progressively stretch muscles, flexibility will increase, and so on. Naturally, you have to be very gradual in applying new, higher levels of physical demand. Otherwise, you could cause injury or over train your body.

For successful muscle development, rest is almost as important as training. Muscles do not progress during the time you are working out, but rather during rest periods that follow. While training, you "tear" the muscles and while resting, you "rebuild" the muscles. Don't get the wrong message, though. Resting without training will not cause progress.

Plateaus during resistance training

You may have heard about plateaus during resistance training, and about techniques of "shocking" the body to avoid plateaus. Proper shocking is actually exposure to new physical stress. Once your body gets used to handling certain types of physical stress, give it something else to work on, something new or forgotten. When it comes to resistance training, you can change the frequency of trainings, type of exercises, number of sets, duration of rest, and so on.

Nevertheless, there is no need to rush changes in training. Apply alterations only when you can see that previous techniques are not giving you satisfactory results any more. If you pay attention, your body will "tell" you when change is needed. If you change variables too fast, you will not have enough time to obtain the full benefit from each technique, and you will exploit too many options too soon. No matter how many techniques you know, and how well you apply them, eventually you will hit a plateau and not progress any more.

It is beyond the scope of this book to give you detailed instructions on a resistance training program. For that, I strongly recommend you seek the assistance of a personal trainer or other specialized source.

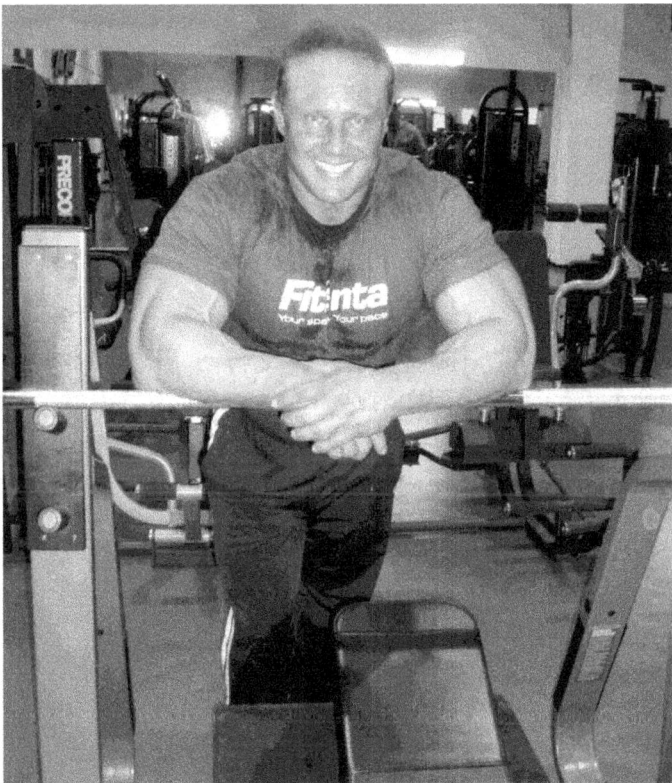

APPENDIX TWO

Don't worry. This will not be tedious sermonizing about healthy eating. Appendix Two presents what you need to know about nutrition that can benefit your day to day fat loss program. The information is useful, straightforward and easy to understand.

NUTRITION

This chapter will explain the basics of nutrition, in general terms relevant for fat loss. To find your exact individual nutritional needs, seek advice from your physician, nutritionist, or other specialists. This is especially the case if you have health problems.

There are six essential nutrients that must be present in optimal balance for proper nutrition every day. We can group them as:

Energy-rich nutrients: *proteins*, *carbohydrates* and *fats*.
Energy-free nutrients: *water*, *vitamins* and *minerals*.

For fat loss purposes, energy consumption is of utmost importance. Therefore, we will be paying the most attention to energy-rich nutrients.

PROTEINS,
ENERGY-RICH NUTRIENTS

Second only to water, proteins are found in the human organism in the highest proportion. They build internal organs, muscles, blood, skin, hair, nails and so on. In addition to primarily being the building material, proteins can be used as an energy source if food intake is too low from carbohydrates and fats. The energy value of proteins is about four calories per gram.

Proteins are built from smaller elements called amino acids. There are about 20 amino acids necessary for building human proteins. Eight of them are called *essential amino acids*, because they cannot be synthesized by the organism itself and must be supplied by food in proper quantity and proportions. Essential amino acids for adults are *isoleucine, leucine, lysine, methionine, phenylalanine, threonine, tryptophan* and *valine*. For infants *arginine* and *histidine* are also essential since their body still cannot produce them.

Types of protein

Based on their essential amino acid content, proteins can be divided into two groups:

- *High quality proteins* (or "complete" proteins) are the proteins with sufficient quantity and proportions of essential amino acids. They are derived from animal sources, including eggs, milk, dairy products, fish and seafood, poultry and meat. At least some of these foods should be present in the diet regularly. When we track the amount of protein consumed, we only count protein from these high quality protein foods towards satisfying our daily protein needs. Foods from these groups are recorded in the fat loss journal for their energy value as well as for the grams of protein they provide.

- *Low quality proteins* (or "incomplete" proteins) are the proteins with insufficient quantity and proportions of essential amino acids. They are derived from non-animal sources, including rice, potatoes, wheat and soy. When we consume these foods, we do not count the protein towards satisfying our daily protein needs. In the fat loss journal, these foods are numerically recorded only for the calories they contain, not grams of protein.

You can combine more than one incomplete protein to make complete proteins. While I have written about this, I myself have not tried it. Rather, I use supplements with essential amino acids if I wish to improve amino acid characteristics of incomplete proteins.

Biological value of protein

Biological value (BV) of protein is a measurement that tells us how well and how quickly our body can use the given protein. BV will be closer to 100 for higher quality protein.

When we talk about high quality proteins that are good enough to be recorded numerically towards satisfying our daily protein needs, we refer to proteins with high BV. To get a sense of the basic idea of the highest quality proteins, you can refer to this listing (values are approximate).

Whey protein	100 BV
Whole egg	95 BV
Cow's milk	85 BV
Chicken and Turkey	80 BV
Fish	75 BV
Beef (other meats)	75 BV

The highest quality protein comes from eggs, milk, and milk products, not poultry, fish and meat. Nature designed eggs and milk to provide the highest quality food for young organisms when their development is the most intensive and sensitive. As vegetarians know very well, and as you can see from the table, there is absolutely no biological need to eat meat in order to satisfy the body's needs for the highest quality proteins.

Vegetarian – To be or not to be

I myself became vegetarian not at all for health reasons, but because eating meat supports inhumane treatment of animals. I do admit I was seriously concerned about how being vegetarian was going to influence me, considering I did not become a vegetarian until I was in my 40's.

Surprisingly, not only do I feel physically better, but also, I don't have any cravings for meat.

You do not have to become a vegetarian to lose fat and feel better. However, if you care about animals and have considered becoming vegetarian for that reason, then go for it. It is much easier than it looks.

Daily protein needs

Opinions on daily protein requirements often differ. Recommended dietary allowances (RDA) state you should consume 0.36 grams of protein per pound of your body weight each day. In the metric system that is 0.8 grams per kilogram of body weight. Such recommendations are for an average physically active, healthy person with a healthy level of body fat. Protein needs are increased during growth, pregnancy, lactation, and some medical conditions. For more specific assistance in assessing your protein needs, seek a professional opinion.

Physically active individuals can consume higher quantities of protein. For athletes in physically demanding sports, depending on the particular sport, daily recommendations are 0.54 to 0.82 grams of high quality protein per pound of body weight. In the metric system that is 1.2 to 1.8 grams per kilogram of body weight.

During my career, I often consumed over one gram of protein per pound of body weight. Yet there is no real need for over-consumption of protein. Exaggerated protein intake does not necessarily mean increased muscle mass, improved sports results or less body fat. In addition, it can cause health problems, especially for individuals with kidney disease.

Daily protein needs (grams of protein per one pound of body weight)	
For non athletes 0.36	For athletes 0.54 to 0.82

Protein consumption

It is commonly believed that humans cannot utilize more than 30-40 grams of protein in one meal for building purposes. If you consume more, it is used for energy or eventually stored as fat. Therefore, in order to satisfy protein requirements optimally, you should eat several smaller protein-rich meals each day.

However, since I stopped competing in bodybuilding and drastically changed my nutrition, these days I do not see any difference in the function or appearance of my body if I increase or decrease my number of high quality protein meals. Maybe I would not have seen any difference if I had done the same even when I competed, but at that time I cared too much about my condition to take a chance. I believe that consuming a high number of protein meals each day is useful for reaching the maximum physical potential of the body. However, in daily life, I question its practical value.

Let us resort to the idea of our original design. Thousands of years ago we could not expect numerous, evenly distributed, high quality protein meals per day. At that time, much the same as wild animals these days, we caught our prey, pigged out, and then had to wait until the next successful hunt. Since this was our daily reality, it is logical to believe that our body is very capable of satisfying its needs with fewer protein meals (we could apply this logic to other nutrients as well). Today we commonly believe in consuming several small protein meals each day. To be on the safe side, follow that recommendation. But, it has happened before and it will happen again: our strong beliefs of today are often proven wrong tomorrow.

For sufficient protein consumption, depending on your individual constitution and preferences, it may be necessary to use food supplements that contain essential amino acids or high quality protein in order to achieve a properly balanced nutritional program.

CARBOHYDRATES, ENERGY-RICH NUTRIENTS

Carbohydrates, also called sugars, are the principal energy source for the body (blood glucose). All molecules of carbohydrates do not have the same structural complexity.

Depending on their structure, they release energy with different dynamics while being broken down in the organism. However, they all have the same energy value of approximately four calories per gram (the same as protein). For fat loss, all that really counts is the number of calories.

Types of carbohydrates

Carbohydrates are usually divided into two basic categories based on the structural complexity of their molecules.

- *Simple carbohydrates* (glucose, fructose and galactose as monosaccharides) are easily digestible because of their simple molecular structure. After consumption they quickly and intensely raise the energy level, that is, the blood glucose level, but only for a short period of time (short-term energy). Soon after, as the energy level drops, hunger and craving for more simple carbohydrates can occur. This is undesirable, especially if on a fat loss program. Do not worry excessively about a possible negative effect, though. Many never feel a sudden energy drop or craving for simple carbohydrates (myself included). Simple carbohydrates are often recommended just before, during or immediately after physical activity for a quick energy boost or successful recovery. They are found mostly in fruits, honey, candies and sweets.

- *Complex carbohydrates* (starch and cellulose as plant, and glycogen as animal polysaccharides) are built by binding simple carbohydrates into a more complex molecular structure. Unlike simple carbohydrates, complex carbohydrates do not release energy quickly and intensively, but rather slowly over a longer period of time (long-term energy). Theoretically, that could prevent the feeling of hunger and food cravings present after the consumption of simple carbohydrates. Polysaccharides are found in rice, potatoes, cereals, seeds and vegetables. In most cases, they are also an excellent source of dietary fiber necessary for proper digestion.

Glycemic index

The glycemic index (GI) ranks carbohydrates according to their effect on our blood glucose levels. Simple carbohydrates have a higher GI, because they cause greater fluctuation in our blood glucose. They quickly and intensely raise the energy level. Complex carbohydrates have a lower GI, because they cause smaller fluctuations in our blood glucose levels. They slowly release energy, spread over a longer period of time. As described before, the GI of carbohydrates could influence your hunger. Other than that, if you are a healthy individual, for your fat loss you can eat any carbohydrate, regardless of GI. They all release the same amount of energy.

Carbohydrate consumption

Daily requirements for carbohydrates mostly depend on the energy level we wish (or need) to generate. It is commonly believed that properly balanced nutrition, including fat loss nutrition, should contain more complex than simple carbohydrates. Personally, I do not notice much practical manifestation of these previously described differences between simple and complex sugars (with high or low GI). In my fat loss journal I record a food rich in carbohydrates only by the total energy it releases (not by structure or grams of carbohydrates), and I eat it based on my preferences rather than such structural characteristics. However, if you have certain medical conditions, in particular diabetes or pre-diabetes, your nutrition should be managed in cooperation with your physician. For fat loss energy deficit will always be required, but your food choices could be necessarily restricted.

Food supplements containing dietary fiber can be very useful, especially for fat loss nutrition. Fat loss nutrition often causes constipation or irregular bowel movements due to intake of smaller amounts of food, and perhaps insufficient total dietary fiber consumed. On the other hand, supplements rich in carbohydrates (or energy in general), that are commonly used for recovery after a workout are not the best choice during fat loss. If you insist on using them, be very careful about your daily energy intake. If you include too much of them, you will not lose fat.

FATS,
ENERGY-RICH NUTRIENTS

Fats, also called lipids, comprise a significant portion of a person's body mass. The percentage of fat is typically somewhat higher in women than men.

Types of fat

In the human organism fats appear in two functional forms:

- *Storage fat* is deposited primarily in the subcutaneous tissue. This fat includes energy storage, and protection for internal organs from various negative influences in the environment (for example, sudden temperature changes and physical injury). When we gain or lose fat, we increase or decrease the quantity of our storage fat.

- *Tissue fat* is a building element of every cell. Its total quantity is mostly constant, contrary to storage fat, whose quantity varies depending on ratios of consumed and spent energy.

Fat in food can be divided into two basic categories:

- *Saturated fats* are primarily found in animal fat.

- *Unsaturated fats* are found in vegetables. They can be further divided into *monounsaturated fats* and *polyunsaturated fats*.

All fats (saturated and unsaturated) are important for proper function and health of the body.

Trans fats

Trans fats are formed by adding hydrogen to liquid vegetable oil, changing it into a form that is solid at room temperature. This chemical process is called hydrogenation. Trans fats are often found in margarine, crackers, candies, baked goods, cookies, snack foods, fried foods, salad dressing, and other highly processed foods. It is recommended to keep consumption of trans fats as low as possible.

Fat consumption

An insufficient amount of fat in nutrition may lead to fat-soluble vitamin deficiencies and cause various health disorders. On the other hand, excessive fat intake may result in fatness due to its high-energy value. One gram of fat yields nine calories, more than twice the calories in one gram of protein or carbohydrates. However, fats do not release energy as readily as carbohydrates. Energy obtained by their breakdown will be longer lasting and lower in intensity.

From the fat loss point of view, all fats release the same energy, regardless of whether they are trans fats, saturated fats or unsaturated fats. Also, excessive energy coming from fats is no more dangerous for fat loss or fat gain than the same amount of excessive energy coming from any other source (proteins, carbohydrates or alcohol). We could go into certain academic discussions about how the body uses energy. The bottom line, though, is that consumed energy is consumed energy, regardless of where it comes from, and spent energy is spent energy, regardless of what you have done to spend it.

When consuming food rich in fats, document in your fat loss journal only the total amount of energy such food releases, and don't worry about what kind or how many grams of fat it contains. As long as you keep control of your total daily caloric intake, you will be fine.

That said, a former client of mine once told me that in his fat loss journal he also records grams of fat. He explained that even though he consciously knows that it is not important, the bad image that fat has for fat loss makes him feel guilty when he consumes too many grams of fat. This is another example of a good use of guilt, similar to using guilt after a day off for more efficient fat loss. It also shows how you can modify a general "rule" (in this case, not to record grams of fat) to create a personalized tool for more effective fat loss.

Even during a very strict fat loss diet, fat will most likely sneak in through some foods, and that is fine. We need fat for proper functioning of our bodies. Also, if you take days off on a regular basis, you should not worry about lack of fat in your fat loss nutrition. However, if you go to the extreme and decide to diet only with fat free foods for a prolonged time, then supplementing with high quality fats is recommended. If you take them, remember to include their caloric value in your daily tracking.

WATER,
AN ENERGY-FREE NUTRIENT

Water is a necessary and unavoidable component of food and living matter. In the body water comes as intracellular (2/3 of total body content) and extracellular fluid (1/3 of total body content). It has many important functions, and only oxygen is more important for immediate survival than water. A person can survive without water for only one to five days depending on the climate, while without food sometimes for more than five weeks. The following are examples of water content in the human organism:

the body of a *newborn* contains about	75% water
the body of an adult *male* (healthy level of body fat) contains about	60% water
the body of an adult *female* (healthy level of body fat) contains about	55% water
the *obese* adult could contain as low as	45% water

Daily water needs

Daily water needs depend on many factors, such as climate, physical activity, body constitution and health. There are indications that an average healthy person should consume about three-quarters of a gallon of water every day. If your energy needs are higher (you are physically more active or you have a large body size), your water needs will be higher. Solid food contains a certain amount of water. For example, fruits and vegetables are about 80 to 90% water. Water contained in solid food also counts towards satisfying our daily water requirements. Water has no energy value for the human organism. No matter how much water you drink, it will not make you fat.

Water is eliminated from the body by urine, feces and perspiration. In extreme situations a person may lose more than two gallons of water a day. This can cause serious dehydration and loss of electrolytes, which have to be replenished by increased drinking and the addition of food supplements.

Carrying water containers around

Although water should not be neglected, you should not burden yourself with dosing or measuring the water you drink. A healthy organism will be able to regulate balance between eliminated and consumed water, unless exposed to severe circumstances of extreme dehydration. Drink when you are thirsty. No need to measure every sip or cart water containers around with you everywhere you go. It is recommended, however, that you increase water intake, and drink smaller amounts of water more frequently, during training or increased physical labor. How much water you need to drink depends on the type and level of physical activity, temperature of environment, perspiration level, and so on. But if you are not exercising (or physically working) hard, no need to increase water intake just because you are in the gym.

Alcohol

Alcohol is very energy-rich and releases seven calories per gram. That makes it basically twice as rich in energy as one gram of protein or carbohydrate, and almost as rich as one gram of fat. Needless to say, excessive consumption of alcohol can compromise the success of your fat loss.

VITAMINS AND MINERALS, ENERGY-FREE NUTRIENTS

Vitamins (which are organic) and minerals (which are inorganic) are crucial substances for proper function of the body. When nutrition is deficient in vitamins or minerals, a number of health disorders may occur. If your diet includes a wide variety of foods, you are probably getting sufficient nutrition. If you are not eating enough foods rich in vitamins and minerals, or if you are dieting for fat loss, vitamin and mineral supplements are recommended.

Regardless of the variety in my own nutrition, I commonly take supplements containing the recommended dietary allowances (RDA) of vitamins and minerals, especially during fat loss, just to be safe. However, many individuals report that they do not see a difference when taking or not taking such supplements. So, check with your nutritionist or other specialized professional to see if your nutrition is vitamin or mineral deficient, or if you actually require additional supplements.

Vitamins and minerals belong to the group of energy-free nutrients. Together with water, they do not release energy when consumed. If you are consuming vitamin or mineral supplements which have other energy-rich nutrients added to their contents, you should consider the energy value of the supplements.

APPENDIX THREE

FREQUENTLY ASKED QUESTIONS

Throughout the various stages of my career, I have been asked a lot of questions about exercise and nutrition related to fat loss. The most relevant and frequent questions are answered in this chapter. If the answer has already been elaborated on in more detail in previous chapters, I have reiterated the bottom line here, and will refer you to the corresponding location in the book.

1. *I eat healthy, so why am I not losing fat?*

    You aren't losing fat because you eat too much so called "healthy food". For fat loss you require an energy deficit, regardless of whether it comes from "healthy" or "unhealthy" eating. However, you should lose fat and, at the same time, maintain or improve your health, so pay attention to proper balance of your nutrition while in energy deficit. But for sheer fat loss, the only thing you need is an energy deficit. For more details see "Eat whatever you want", page 63-67.

2. *Do I need to be on a low carb diet to lose fat?*

    No, you do not. The principal energy source for the body is blood sugar, or glucose. Even if you consume zero carbohydrates, the body will create glucose from other nutrients, so there is no point in "counting" carbs. That is a waste of time. Count calories instead, and you will lose fat! When it comes to fat loss alone, low carb diets are nothing but another media-created diversion to proper thinking about fat loss. How many copies of their fat loss-related magazines would they sell, or what kind of audience for their TV shows would they have, if instead they told the simple truth? "You will lose fat only by energy deficit, and that's all you need".

3. *I hardly eat anything, so how come I still cannot lose weight?*

If that is true (and usually it is not), the reason may be that the body has adapted to a lower energy intake. To increase the energy requirements of your body, start exercising. In reality, though, you are eating much more than "hardly anything". People often do not see, or do not wish to see how much food they actually consume. A snack here, a bite there, plus a few drinks, and there you are, the calorie count is far above your daily requirement. That's why an accurate fat loss journal is valuable help. If you record everything you consume, you will have exact facts and you will not even ask this question anymore.

4. *Why are snacks so dangerous for fat loss?*

They are not dangerous at all. They are perceived as dangerous simply because people lose track of how many small snacks they have had during the day. No matter how many calories a small bite of something has, it will not be enough to make a person fat by itself. What makes people fat is one small bite after the other all day long. If you can limit yourself when it comes to snacks, you will be just fine.

5. *Which foods are not fattening?*

Some foods are lower in calories than others. But all foods containing proteins, carbohydrates or fats, release a certain amount of energy, and that energy accumulates during the day. If your energy intake is greater than your energy expenditure you will gain fat, regardless of the foods you eat. For more details see "Pick foods with fewer calories", page 173-176.

6. *Do I need to eat food high in calories in order to get fatter?*

If you are genetically a skinny person, or you have lost fat due to a proper fat loss program, you may want to gain a certain amount of fat. If so, you do not need to eat cheesecake, ice cream, cookies, or other high-calorie foods in order to get fatter. The principle is the same as with losing fat, but it just goes in the opposite direction.

To get fatter you have to create an energy surplus, irrespective of the type of food. However, it will be much easier and often tastier to create an energy surplus if you eat high-calorie food.

7. *What foods increase my sexual potency without making me fat?*

I have no idea, but please let me know if you find out. However, I can tell you two things. Nothing will make you fat if you don't eat too much of it. And, if you eat too much, not only will you get fat, but also with a full stomach you will not be a Tarzan in the bedroom.

8. *Is losing fat different between men and women?*

There are no essential differences. Both men and women require an energy deficit to lose fat, and to achieve it they should eat less and be physically active. However, women naturally have a bit more fat than men, therefore generally they will not be able, nor should they try, to drop their body fat percentage as low as men can in extreme cases.

9. *Is it necessary to avoid salt when trying to lose fat?*

Salt does not have any calories. Therefore, it will not increase fat deposits even if consumed excessively. However, if your salt intake is high, you can look fatter, bloated and even gain some weight, not because you have gained more fat, but due to water retention. For more details see "Water retention - Salt's fault", page 94-96.

10. Is vegetarian nutrition lower in calories and better for fat loss?

Vegetarian nutrition does not automatically imply lower calorie intake than conventional nutrition. Vegetarians also have to control their energy intake in order to create an energy deficit and lose fat. Switching to vegetarianism will not give you an obvious upper hand with fat loss, but it could contribute to your overall well-being and most certainly will be more humane to animals.

11. I only eat once a day, so why am I still fat?

It is a mistake to eat only once (or twice) a day, while starving and being physically passive through the rest of the day. In spite of only one meal consumed, this is an excellent short cut to muscle loss and fat gain. Consume several low-calorie, properly balanced meals each day. For more information see "Eat more small meals each day", page 176-179.

12. What kind of diet do I have to use so I do not gain fat ever again once I stop losing fat?

To lose fat you have to consume less energy than your body needs. You will be lean (or keep your current body weight) as long as you maintain the balance between energy in and energy out. When you hear stories about people who used certain diets, lost fat, and never gained it back again, know this. They did not gain fat back because they kept their energy intake low enough, not because they lost fat by way of some particular diet or exercise. For more details see "Lose it and keep it lean", page 98-101.

13. Do I have to eat more in order to speed up my metabolism so I can lose fat?

This is one of my favorites! Let me make sure I understand this right. (1) We know beyond a doubt that we get fat by consuming too much energy, and to lose fat we have to consume less energy than we need. (2) The person asking this question is not losing fat at the current energy intake, but in order to lose fat, wants to consume even more energy.

No, of course you do not have to eat more in order to lose fat! You just have to eat less and be a bit hungry. If you are hungry, you are probably burning fat. If you are hungry but not burning fat, then you are not hungry enough. Simple and logical reasoning leads to the best conclusions. Is it logical to eat more to lose fat? Have you ever heard an opposing question, "Do I have to eat less in order to slow down my metabolism so I can gain fat?" Don't fear slow metabolism, fear instead a fast feeding hand.

14. *On nutritional labels, what does sugar mean? Isn't sugar another name for carbohydrates?*

Sugar is indeed just a common name for carbohydrates. However, on nutritional labels, in the section for carbohydrates, sugar commonly refers to a group of added sweeteners, such as refined or table sugar, honey, rice syrup and so forth. These substances are added to the product to create a sweeter taste, preferred by consumers. For fat loss it is all the same, one gram of carbohydrates equals four calories, regardless of whether you call it sugar or not. Do not fear "sugar" in your fat loss. Fear "overeating" and "energy surplus".

15. *Is it true that some foods contain enzymes that promote fat loss?*

It is popular to talk about the various enzymes or other chemical constituents of food, particularly in view of fat loss. No single food contains any significant amount of enzymes or anything else that obviously contributes to fat loss, and excessive consumption of such a food or product is not justifiable. When it comes to fat loss, don't even bother searching for exotic solutions. You need only one thing: energy deficit.

16. *Is there any truth in advertising for fat loss products?*

Possibly there is. If they are saying you need to exercise, be hungry and work hard to lose fat, and really do not need their product, they are not lying at all. The biggest lies are promises that you will accomplish fat loss quickly and easily, that you will lose fat and keep it off, or guarantees that you will see results after only using their product. For more details see "Fat loss products", page 192-205.

17. *What food supplements or products can I use to quickly lose fat or gain muscle?*

Any legal product should have at least some scientifically proven reason for its existence. When you take such a product, you are only slightly, if at all, increasing your potential to reach your goal. For losing fat or gaining muscle, the most important components are adequate exercise, nutrition and lifestyle. Every process of improving your body condition requires knowledgeable effort over a prolonged period of time. The saying, "Anything worth having does not come easily" applies well to fat loss and muscle development. For more details see "Fat loss products", page 192-205.

18. What is the difference in effectiveness between legal and illegal products (doping)?

Illegal products (doping), if taken with proper training, nutrition and lifestyle, are by far more effective than legal products, especially in developing muscle mass, but much less effective for losing fat. If such illegal products are taken without sufficient training, nutrition and an appropriate lifestyle, the desired result will not come. These products do not produce results by themselves, which is a common misconception. They just enable you to keep benefiting from your efforts and hard work a bit more (not indefinitely) than you would if progressing in a strictly natural way or with legal products alone. Regardless, doping is better avoided, if for no other reason, than simply because it is illegal.

19. Is there a difference between fat loss and weight loss?

Fat loss refers precisely to fat reduction and in most cases will be accompanied by weight loss, too. Weight loss is obviously a reduction of body weight but could be completely unrelated to fat loss. For more details see "Weight loss vs. fat loss", page 35-37.

20. How many people actually reach their fat loss goal?

Not many people successfully achieve their fat loss goal, and out of those that do most gain fat back shortly after they finish their diet. Even though the rate of success is low, that should not discourage you. Be aware of the fat loss facts, and use them to make yourself stronger and more determined to achieve and maintain your leaner condition.

21. Can I turn fat into muscle?

You can't. Rather, you most likely need to get rid of fat first, and then try to develop muscles. You can also reverse the order, by first developing additional muscles and then getting rid of undesired fat deposits. If you choose to do it that way, then during the muscle development phase and before losing fat, the body will look even fatter than before. Also, the actual effects of the muscle development process will be harder to detect, because the fat deposits will distort an objective evaluation. You may think you are developing more muscle, but in fact you are just getting fatter. In most cases it is better to reduce fat deposits first, and then try to develop additional muscle mass. For more details see "Weight loss vs. fat loss", page 35-37 and "Anaerobic physical activities", page 219-223.

22. How do I get firm buttocks and thighs?

If you have this problem, get rid of the excess fat. The cause of the sagging or soft appearance is not poor muscle firmness, but rather the amount of fat that covers the muscles. For both "big and heavy" body types as well as "thin and light" ones, the solution is pretty much the same. Lose fat. Sometimes, for the best results, I also recommend you try to develop some muscle mass, after or maybe even before you lose fat. For more details see "Spot fat reduction – Wishful thinking", page 87-92.

23. *I want to tone, firm and define my body – do I need to lose fat too?*

To tone, firm and define your body you most likely need to lose fat. Individuals with "thin and light" body types will commonly use such terms because they think fat loss does not apply to them since they don't weigh 300 lbs. Such body types, regardless of their smaller size and body mass, can still have an excessive amount of fat. That is what gives them their soft and undefined look. The solution is the reduction of excessive fat deposits in combination with muscle development.

24. *How can I lose weight before summer?*

This is only possible if summer is not too close, and the fat deposits are not too big. Apply the rules described in this book, and you will lose fat. However, the question indicates the wrong approach. When you decide to improve the condition of your body, your motivation should not be this summer, but all summers year after year. You should have long-term goals, which will enable you to generate a permanent motivation for adopting a leaner lifestyle. "Important dates" can make you more motivated, and snap you out of a bad routine, and that is better than nothing. Sometimes we do great things for the wrong reasons.

25. *Am I on the right track to lose fat by doing what I am doing now?*

If you are at the beginning of your fat loss process, and results are not obvious yet, ask yourself a question, "Will I get where I want to be by doing what I am doing now?" Be realistic in your answer, not delusional and unrealistically optimistic. A fat loss quantum leap does not exist. You cannot win a "fat loss lottery" and one day wake up lean. Being "realistically optimistic" is very good, but if you jump from a skyscraper hoping you will grow wings before you hit the ground, that is "delusional" and "unrealistically optimistic". I know this example sounds ridiculous, but many people hope for almost equally unreal results when losing fat.

If you have been dieting for a while and are achieving results, keep doing whatever you are doing as long as you are losing fat and feeling good. Once progress stops, then changes are needed. See "How many calories?" page 116-125.

26. I hope I only need to lose 10 pounds to look my best. Does this seem right?

In my experience people usually greatly underestimate the amount of fat they have to lose. For example, if you think you will be at your desired body condition with 10 pounds of less fat, it will actually take you 20 or even more pounds to get there. In some cases your original expectation can be completely accurate, but that happens very rarely.

27. Do I need a training partner to lose fat?

A good training partner can be very helpful to keep you motivated, especially if you have similar goals. If knowledgeable, a partner can also teach you a lot about training and nutrition. On the other hand, I strongly urge you to stay away from training buddies that are lazy, flaky, not motivated or without a goal. If you incorporate them into your fat loss program, they will virtually destroy your chances of success. They will gradually corrode all of your positive intentions and actions, just like placing a rotten apple next to a healthy one.

However, if you do not have a good training partner, you really do not need one. Often we hear excuses like, "I was doing just fine until my friend stopped doing it with me." With this kind of attitude you would not have finished, even if your friend had not quit! The bottom line is: fat loss is a one-person job, and you are the only person who can do it.

28. *Should I keep a fat loss journal?*

That is optional, but highly recommended, because a fat loss journal will be a tremendous support. It will provide facts and data that you need. Without a journal you will have only a vague idea or, even worse, no idea at all what is going on with your fat loss. Even after 25 years of manipulating body fat, when I am attempting serious fat loss, I keep a journal. For more information see "Fat loss journal - Navigate by compass, not by breeze", page 126-132.

29. *How reliable are various methods of measuring body fat percentage?*

Every body fat measuring method used in sports and recreation is more or less accurate "guessing". Sometimes such "guessing" can be really accurate, especially as technology progresses and more accurate methods become available. But some methods can give ridiculously wrong results. For instance, at the end of one of my fat loss programs one method showed me 17% and 19% body fat respectively (measured twice, within a few minutes), while immediately after, measurement by skin folds indicated 5.4%. I was highly conditioned at that time, so the results of 17% and 19% were obviously wrong. The method that provided the wrong results was based on the same technology as home scales that provide body fat percentage evaluation. This is one of the reasons why I prefer measuring body fat by skinfolds. Such methods are "robust", simple, accessible and logical; the thicker your skin is, the fatter you are. For more details see "Determining fatness", page 38-44.

30. *Why do we get fatter with age, or after an active athletic career?*

The human organism decreases its energy requirements with age. Besides that, as we get older we are usually physically less active. That is especially the case with athletes after a competitive career. If for many years you were an athlete on a diet with a high energy intake, adjust your nutrition promptly after you stop competing. If calorie intake is not reduced adequately, getting fatter is inevitable.

31. *Why does my body shape change throughout the day (I get softer, flatter and bloated) even though I am on a strict fat loss program?*

Noticeable changes in body shape are possible over the course of only a few hours. The intensity of these changes varies individually, but is more obvious if your body is in better shape (has less fat). Body shape is usually the best in the morning hours, while it can noticeably worsen during the day. Such changes are related to water retention and the balance of fluid in the body. If you stay on your fat loss diet, these problems should not worry you, because they are temporary and do not mean you actually have become fatter. Tomorrow morning you will look good again.

32. Why did I not get my period? Is it because of training and diet?

A strict diet and exhausting trainings can cause menstrual cycle disorders or fluctuations. According to some sources, a woman will lose her period if her body fat percentage drops below about 10%, and a man will lose his period if his body fat percentage drops below 5%. That reference to a man losing his period was a test to see if you are paying attention.

Back to being serious now, when any menstrual cycle disorder occurs, you should seek medical attention, and if exposed to rigorous diet and exercise, change your conditioning program. That is, eat more well-balanced food, and reduce physical activity.

33. Why do I gain weight during my period?

Just before the period your body weight may increase by several pounds because of water retention, but after the period your weight should return to the previous level. This phenomenon has nothing to do with gaining additional fat. Also, some medications may increase water retention in the body.

34. *How do I lose weight and get in shape after pregnancy?*

While pregnant and during breastfeeding, you should not try to lose fat. You should also not use such conditions as excuses for exaggerated eating, either. It is considered that during pregnancy the mother needs an average of only about 300 calories more each day than what her energy needs were prior to pregnancy. To put this in perspective, this is the energy from about two or three apples. However, do not count calories while pregnant or breastfeeding. Your body will tell you what it needs, so listen to it.

Be aware of priorities. Even if you gain extra fat while pregnant or breastfeeding, that is better than not having enough food. When pregnancy and breastfeeding are over, if you wish to lose fat, go about your fat loss like anybody else and as described in this book. To be on the safe side, before you start your fat loss, consult your physician.

35. *I have a hormonal imbalance. What do I do to lose fat?*

Another one of my favorite excuses people use to not lose fat! Such a disorder may require your fat loss efforts to be a bit greater, but it cannot stop you from losing fat. Simply put, you might have to eat a bit less food in order to create a sufficient energy deficit and fat loss, compared to the amount of food that you could eat if you did not have a hormonal imbalance. If you adhere to the principles presented in this book the result will not fail. In the case of a hormonal disorder, it is necessary to consult your physician – but for medical reasons only, not to find out whether or not you can lose fat. You can. For more information, see "What makes us fat?" page 45-48.

36. How much effort is required for maintaining a good figure?

Maintaining a good figure usually requires less effort than accomplishing it. How much effort it requires to maintain your body shape also depends on the level where you want to keep it. Conceptually, to maintain 80% of your "perfect" figure takes about 20% effort, whereas to keep or to achieve the remaining 20% of your "perfect" figure requires the remaining 80% effort. If you settle for a little less than your "perfect" body shape, it should not be very difficult to maintain or even achieve it. For more details see "Lose it and keep it lean", page 98-101.

37. Which resistance training exercises are for gaining muscle and which are for losing fat?

Resistance training exercises should not be divided in such a way. You have to select exercises that are the most suitable for you. Then use them during a muscle gain and fat loss period. During fat loss you use the same exercises, but with a bit lighter weights and more repetitions. That will reduce the possibility of injury because the body gets weaker during fat loss, especially after significant body weight has been reduced. For more details see "Anaerobic physical activities", page 219-223.

38. Is it possible to significantly change the basic shape of muscles?

No it is not. If properly applied, weights and machines used in fitness and bodybuilding workouts can change the look of your muscles more effectively than any other method of physical training. With proper resistance training you can make your muscles bigger, more pronounced, stronger, faster, more powerful and resilient, but unfortunately nothing can change the basic shape of muscles.

For instance, if thighs tend to look "square", they will always have the same basic shape, regardless of whether they are extremely developed or not developed at all. Another popular example is "short and pointy" biceps. Regardless of the workout routine, the basic shape will stay the same.

If you do not like your basic muscle shape, you can make other positive changes and at least partially compensate for what you do not like. What can often severely distort the picture of the real basic shape of your muscles is the layer of fat that covers them. Before you draw any conclusions, get rid of the excessive fat deposits.

39. *How can training lift, enhance and/or shape a woman's breasts?*

Various exercises can be used to train chest muscles. However, a woman's breasts are not just muscles, but other types of tissue as well, including fatty tissue and glandular tissue. Therefore, in this context, no physical exercise will significantly contribute to the whole breast area, shaping it to your satisfaction. Rather, primarily muscles will be shaped. If you are unhappy with your current breast shape, either make your peace with it or resort to cosmetic surgery.

40. *How do I pick the right fitness center for fat loss?*

Almost any contemporary fitness center should be just fine. When choosing which one, consider the location, commute, the variety of equipment, the size of the physical space, how many people attend, and so on. Your evaluation of these factors is entirely personal to you. However, purely from the fat loss point of view, any gym could serve this purpose very well, even with modest equipment. It is not what you find in the gym, but what you bring with you to the gym that will make a difference in the success of your workout. For more details see "Must I go to a fitness center?" page 69-73.

41. *Why do I "suddenly" gain weight when I start working out with weights?*

This could happen because of the initial development of your muscles under training. Even if you lose some fat during that time and now have a smaller total body volume, your weight can increase due to the greater specific mass of muscle tissue compared to fat.

Sudden initial weight gain due to muscle development will be limited and should not persist especially if it happens during fat loss. If it does, your body weight is most likely increased due to fat gain not muscle development. For more information see "Weight loss vs. fat loss", page 35-37 and "Determining fatness", page 38-44.

42. *Will working out give me visible veins?*

Any physical strain increases the requirement for blood supply. During that time you could experience temporary "surfacing" of blood vessels. But when you stop the physical activity, they should go back to their usual condition. Permanent changes are possible after very strenuous workouts over a long period of time. However, visibility of veins is mostly a result of your particular genetics rather than exercise.

A similar phenomenon may be a consequence of "skin thinning" due to fat loss. Skin with a thinner layer of fat underneath will show more blood vessels. Then if you become fatter again, your blood vessels will not be as obvious any more.

43. *Does the penis get larger if you lose fat?*

Your penis will not actually grow if you lose fat, but it will stick out farther as fat from your stomach and surrounding areas retreats during fat loss. That will make your penis look and perform like it actually is longer. Sometimes I am also asked if the penis will shrink due to fat loss. It will not.

44. *Is it true that muscles sag and become extremely soft after you stop training with weights, even worse than if you had never exercised?*

As an exaggerated analogy, who will have worse breath and periodontal health, someone who has never brushed, or someone who hasn't brushed recently? Apply the same reasoning to muscle training. After you stop exercising with weights or in any other way, muscles will lose some of their characteristics, but they will always look and function better than muscles that have never been trained.

45. *Do I need to wear plastic work-out suits while exercising so I can sweat more in order to speed up my fat loss?*

No, you do not. Wearing plastic work-out suits will only increase sweating, not fat loss. Fat loss will happen as a result of energy deficit, not dehydration. For more information see "Dehydration is not fat loss", page 96-98.

46. *How much body weight will I lose overnight?*

Your morning weight will almost always be lower than the night weight recorded before going to bed. That is, of course, if you do not eat or drink during the night. During the night you lose fluid by breathing, sweating and using the toilet. How much lighter you will be in the morning depends on several factors, like body type and size, nutrition, temperature and so on. I usually lose about one pound per night.

This information is particularly useful for athletes in weight-division sports. If you are losing weight to fit into a specific weight division, test how much weight you commonly lose overnight, so you can more accurately plan your body weight adjustment. Keep in mind that significant weight reduction, especially by dehydration will cause you to have reduced physical capabilities.

47. How come I am not losing weight when I drink only shakes?

I hear this question very often. No matter what you consume (shakes, drinks, liquid or solid food, supplements, or other) if it contains energy, you will not lose weight if you consume too much of it. Therefore, decrease the size or number of shakes you drink and you will lose fat and reduce your body weight.

48. How can I lose fat without giving up fatty and sweet foods?

Figuratively speaking, an energy-reduced diet makes up at least 70% of successful fat loss. If you are serious about getting into shape, you should definitely control your food intake. For example, you can easily eat an average sized chocolate bar (about 3-4 ounces), which has over 500 calories. However, you will have to run for 45 minutes at a speed of nine miles per hour to burn that many calories. So, the choice is yours.

These numbers may vary, but the principle is still the same. No amount or type of physical exercise will ever be able to use all energy gained by excessive consumption. Energy reduced nutrition is the king of successful fat loss. But you do not have to give up on fatty and sweet foods. Just have less of them. Energy deficit, not choice of food, is the key to fat loss.

In life you always have to give up one thing to get another. It is for you to decide if you would rather give up a bit of food, or the quality of the rest of your life that is compromised by your fatness. Consider the bottom line. You enjoy food in total no more than an hour each day. Is that one hour of enjoyment worth sacrificing the enjoyment of the remaining 23 hours?

> **IT COMES DOWN TO THIS:**
> *Is one hour a day of*
> ***- taste -***
> *in your mouth worth sacrificing the quality of*
> ***- life -***
> *of the remaining 23 hours because of fatness?*

INDEX

A

B

C

D

P

Q

R

S

T

SPONSOR:

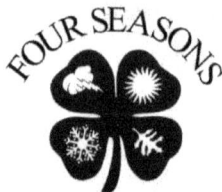

ABOUT NEVEN ČORAK

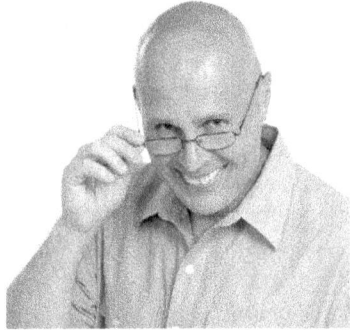

Neven was born in Zagreb, Croatia and moved to the United States in 2001. In his youth he was heavily influenced by his father Josip Čorak, a world-class Olympic wrestler, and participated successfully in many sports, including track-and-field, swimming, wrestling and karate.

Later Neven became involved in the sport of bodybuilding, for which he won numerous awards and competitions. His most significant accomplishments include first place at the European Championship ILBB in 1993, second place as Mr. Universe NABBA in 2005, and first place in the World Cup BNFF-WFF in 2006.

After winning his first European medal in bodybuilding in 1991, Neven brought his expertise to the citizens of Croatia through the media. He became producer and director of two TV shows: "Body Heat" (HRT Croatian Radio Television) and "Beautiful Body by Neven Čorak" (OTV Open Television). Neven appeared in numerous television shows, advertisements and musical videos. In addition he was featured as a columnist in many Croatian magazines, played a role in the movie "Nausikaja", and co-hosted over 80 radio broadcasts.

While engaged in his professional and athletic pursuits, Neven served at various times as head trainer, manager, director, owner and member of the Board of Directors of numerous sports, fitness, and recreation centers in Croatia.

Neven is the published author of eight books in Croatia on

the topic of fitness, bodybuilding, fat loss and nutrition, including *Fitness & Bodybuilding* (2001) and *Basics of Nutrition for Sports and Recreation* (2000).The book you are reading is his first publication intended for the American market.

Neven retired from competitive bodybuilding in 2007. In addition to earlier training in medical nutrition, he holds bachelor and master degrees in Kinesiology, and is currently completing his doctorate work. He resides with his family in Denver, Colorado, where he remains professionally involved in sport and fitness, as well as real estate.

For more information about Neven, please visit:

www.neven-corak.com

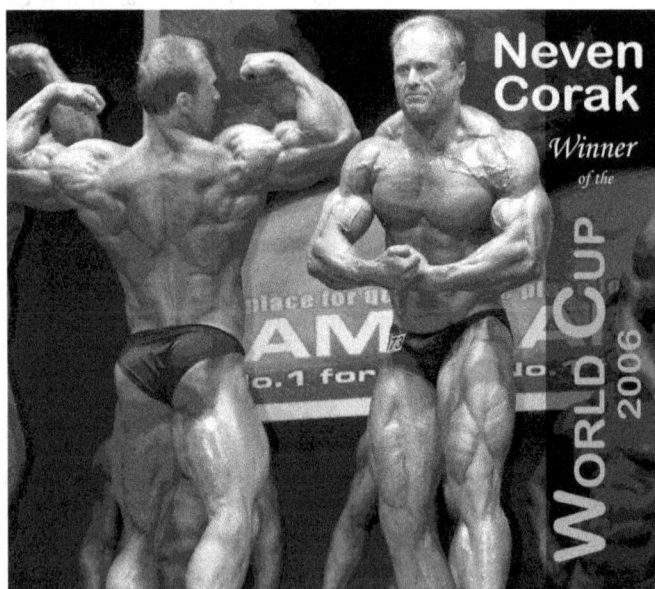

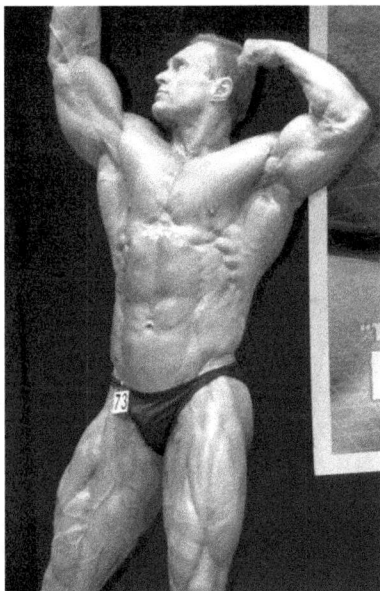

Neven Čorak
Mr. Universe 2005
2nd place

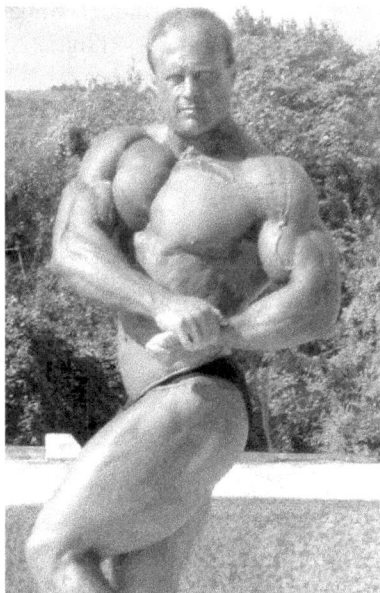

Neven Čorak
World Cup 2006
1st place

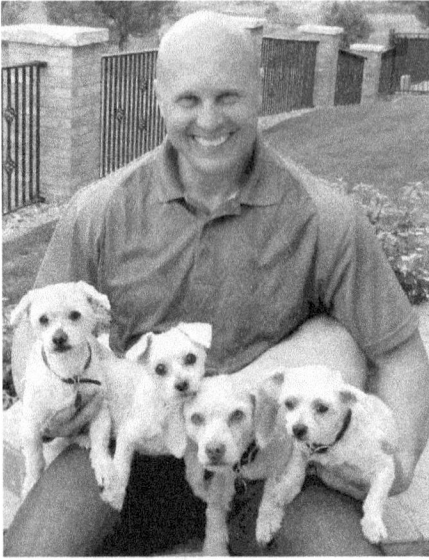

Neven with
Hektor, Astra,
Copper and Casper
(April, 2012)

Neven with Raquel, Anna, Joseph and Claudia
(June, 2014)

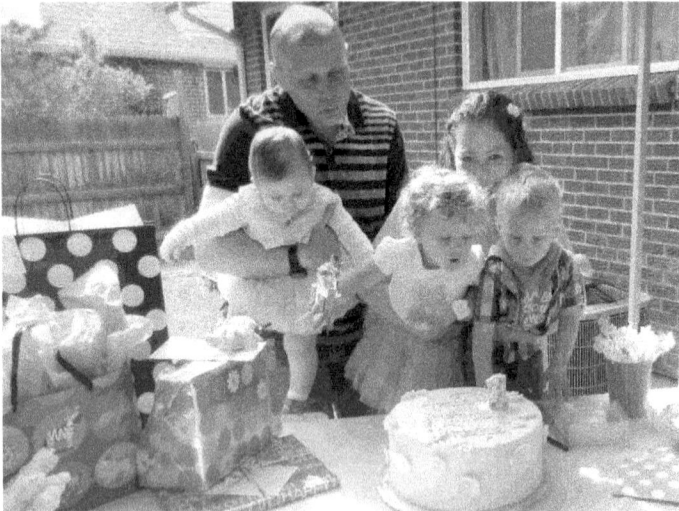